HEALTH CARE

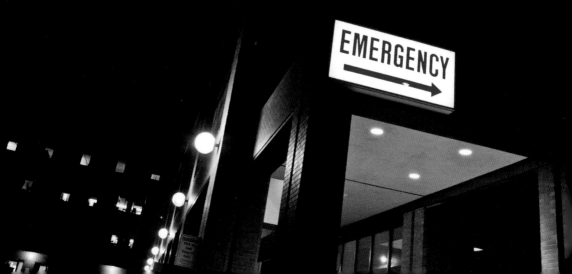

EMERGENCY →

CONTEMPORARY ISSUES

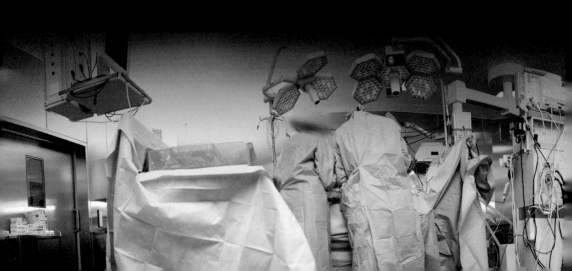

CONTEMPORARY ISSUES

HEALTH CARE

MARK R. WHITTINGTON

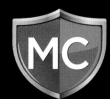

MASON CREST
450 Parkway Drive, Suite D, Broomall, Pennsylvania 19008
(866) MCP-BOOK (toll-free) • www.masoncrest.com

Printed and bound in the United States of America.

CPSIA Compliance Information: Batch #CCRI2019.
For further information, contact Mason Crest at 1-866-MCP-Book.

First printing
1 3 5 7 9 8 6 4 2

ISBN (hardback) 978-1-4222-4393-0
ISBN (series) 978-1-4222-4387-9
ISBN (ebook) 978-1-4222-7408-8

Library of Congress Cataloging-in-Publication Data

Interior and cover design: Torque Advertising + Design
Production: Michelle Luke

Publisher's Note: Websites listed in this book were active at the time of publication. The publisher is not responsible for websites that have changed their address or discontinued operation since the date of publication. The publisher reviews and updates the websites each time the book is reprinted.

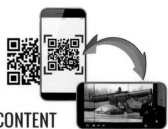

QR CODES AND LINKS TO THIRD-PARTY CONTENT

You may gain access to certain third-party content ("Third-Party Sites") by scanning and using the QR Codes that appear in this publication (the "QR Codes"). We do not operate or control in any respect any information, products, or services on such Third-Party Sites linked to by us via the QR Codes included in this publication, and we assume no responsibility for any materials you may access using the QR Codes. Your use of the QR Codes may be subject to terms, limitations, or restrictions set forth in the applicable terms of use or otherwise established by the owners of the Third-Party Sites. Our linking to such Third-Party Sites via the QR Codes does not imply an endorsement or sponsorship of such Third-Party Sites or the information, products, or services offered on or through the Third-Party Sites, nor does it imply an endorsement or sponsorship of this publication by the owners of such Third-Party Sites.

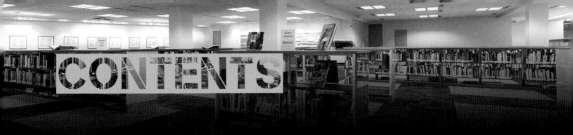

CONTENTS

KEY ICONS TO LOOK FOR:

Words to Understand: These words with their easy-to-understand definitions will increase the reader's understanding of the text while building vocabulary skills.

Sidebars: This boxed material within the main text allows readers to build knowledge, gain insights, explore possibilities, and broaden their perspectives by weaving together additional information to provide realistic and holistic perspectives.

Educational videos: Readers can view videos by scanning our QR codes, providing them with additional educational content to supplement the text. Examples include news coverage, moments in history, speeches, iconic sports moments, and much more!

Text-Dependent Questions: These questions send the reader back to the text for more careful attention to the evidence presented there.

Research Projects: Readers are pointed toward areas of further inquiry connected to each chapter. Suggestions are provided for projects that encourage deeper research and analysis.

Series Glossary of Key Terms: This back-of-the-book glossary contains terminology used throughout this series. Words found here increase the reader's ability to read and comprehend higher-level books and articles in this field.

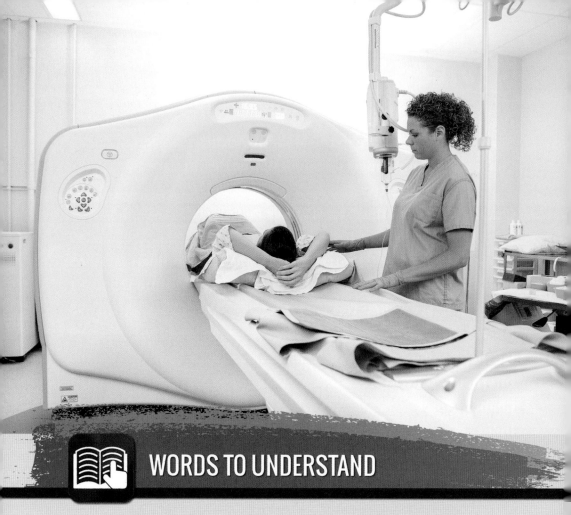

telemedicine—the use of computer technology to allow doctors to treat patients at great distances.

internet of things—devices such as medical sensors that are connected by the internet to allow the distribution of information.

stem cells—cells that can be manipulated to transform into any human body cell.

genetic therapy—a technique that alters the human genome to eliminate diseases.

heroic measures—artificial or emergency health care measures, including the use of machinery, that are intended to revive a dying person.

HEALTH CARE IN THE MODERN WORLD

The state of modern health care can be said to be the best of times and the worst of times. Medical science is rolling out treatments for diseases that just a few years ago would have seemed like science fiction. Healthier living, eating more sensibly, engaging in physical exercise, and avoiding tobacco products have also contributed to a decrease in diseases. The American Cancer Society recently noted that cancer deaths have declined 26 percent from their peak in 1991. "This decline translates to nearly 2.4 million deaths averted during this time period," the ACS stated in a press release.[1]

Unfortunately, these medical advances have been accompanied by a huge increase in the cost of health care, which has made it unaffordable to many Americans. Not only is the cost of medical treatment increasing, but so are deductibles—the amount a person must pay out of pocket before their insurance will being to cover their treatment. These trends have caused some people to skip needed health care services, which puts their health and well-being at risk. "For individuals with insurance cover-age, health care costs were still an issue," writes Jacqueline LaPointe. "Almost 17 percent of individuals who said they or their relatives have avoided care were enrolled in Medicare or Medicaid, 29 percent were covered by plans offered by the private market, and 22 percent had employer-sponsored insurance."[2]

A solution to this problem has proven elusive. The Patient Protection and Affordable Care Act, passed by Congress in 2010, was designed in part to address the exploding costs of health care and, at the same time, to expand access to health insurance. However, the legislation—popularly known as Obamacare—has both supporters and detractors. Supporters note that it succeeded in providing health insurance to over 20 million people who

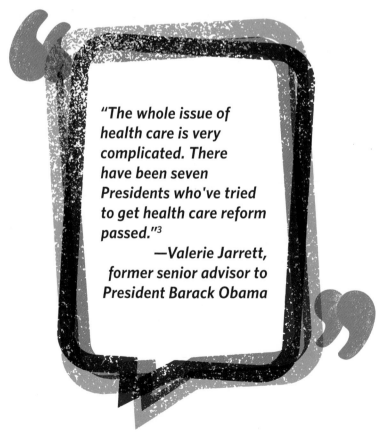

"The whole issue of health care is very complicated. There have been seven Presidents who've tried to get health care reform passed."[3]
—Valerie Jarrett, former senior advisor to President Barack Obama

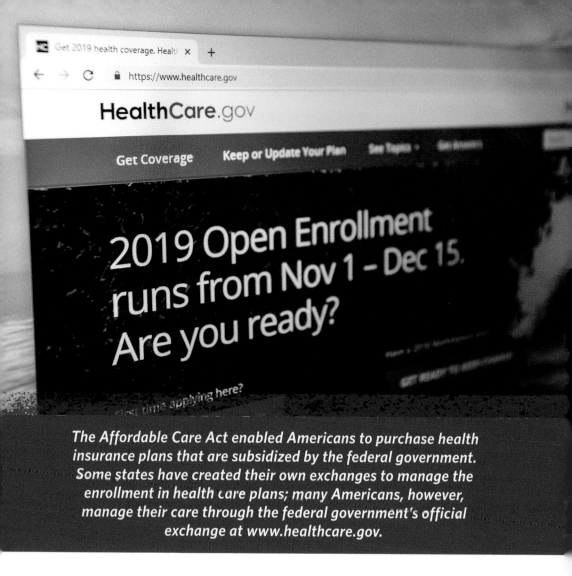

The Affordable Care Act enabled Americans to purchase health insurance plans that are subsidized by the federal government. Some states have created their own exchanges to manage the enrollment in health care plans; many Americans, however, manage their care through the federal government's official exchange at www.healthcare.gov.

previously had no health insurance. However, conservative groups like the Heritage Foundation argue that the legislation has caused insurance premiums to increase, not decrease as some legislators had promised. In a March 2018 study, Heritage Foundation scholars Edmund Haislmaier and Doug Badger found that "premiums for individual coverage more than doubled between 2013 and 2017, and rates rose again in 2018."[4]

Some politicians, notably Senator Bernie Sanders of Vermont, have proposed the creation of a universal health care system in the United States, funded by the government, similar to the public health care systems of Canada and Great Britain. Such proposals have, in turn, sparked huge political battles concerning the desirability of such a

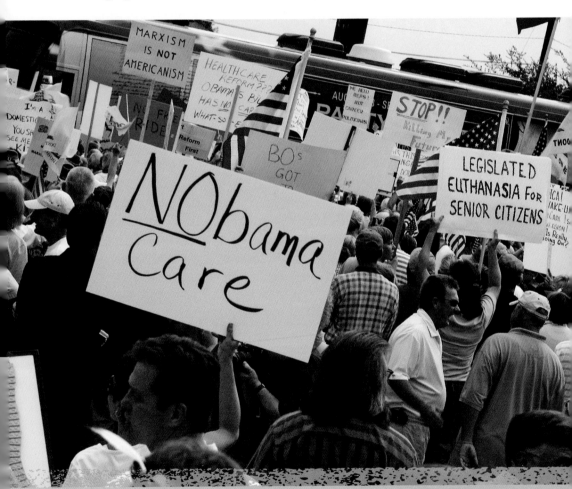

In December 2018, a federal judge in Texas ruled that the Affordable Care Act's mandate requiring people to buy health insurance was unconstitutional.

system and whether it would actually work in a country of more than 325 million people.

One of the more immediate problems facing modern health care has been the skyrocketing cost of drugs in the American market. Some of those drugs, such as insulin, are so necessary for certain groups of people that they will literally die if they can't have them. Yet, if a person is not covered by insurance or has a policy with a high deductible, these lifesaving drugs are often very expensive.

Drug price inflation has sparked off another controversy, with one group of politicians and activists accusing the pharmaceutical companies of placing their profits over the lives and health of their customers. They demand that drug prices be regulated and controlled in the United States, as is the case in many other countries. Others maintain that the drug market's own structure has caused these price

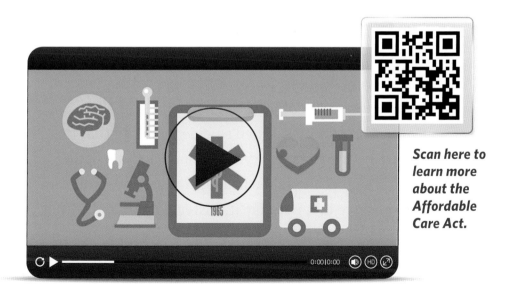

Scan here to learn more about the Affordable Care Act.

spikes and have called for reforms in this area.

Another issue in the United States is related to end-of-life care for those who are terminally ill. Relatives and friends of ailing patients often face the gut-wrenching decision of whether to keep an ailing relative or loved one alive using **heroic measures,** or whether to simply render palliative care and allow nature to take its course.

A process known as assisted suicide takes the matter one step further. Systems have been set up in some countries and even certain US states that allow doctors to painlessly but efficiently put their patients to death. The theory is that certain diseases such as cancer can cause so much pain and take away so much quality of life that when death is inevitable anyway, it is best to speed the process along, painlessly and with dignity. This practice gained notoriety during the 1990s through the work of Dr. Jack Kevorkian, an advocate of assisted suicide who used a machine that he invented to painlessly hasten the deaths of over 130 terminally ill patients. Kevorkian's activities sparked a great deal of controversy, court battles, and an eventual jail term for second-degree murder in 1999.

Those who oppose assisted suicide maintain that the procedure goes against everything that a doctor should be about. Doctors should be healers, they argue, and should preserve life, not take it. Instead, opponents often advocate for improved hospice care, in which a patient's final days can be managed with dignity and their pain mitigated. Medical advances are rendering many diseases

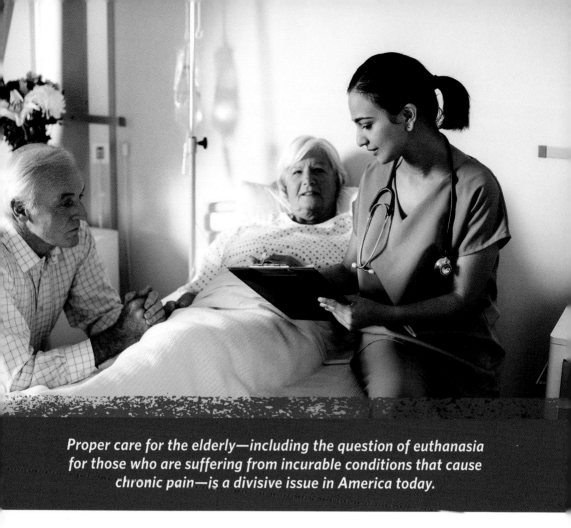

Proper care for the elderly—including the question of euthanasia for those who are suffering from incurable conditions that cause chronic pain—is a divisive issue in America today.

once thought to be incurable to be at least treatable, giving years of life to patients who before had little to look forward to but an early and often painful death.

Medical marijuana has become another issue facing policy makers and the medical professions. Recreational use of marijuana use has been restricted by federal and state governments since the 1930s. However, over the past two decades researchers have recognized that marijuana has some legitimate medical uses as well. In some forms, the drug can reduce the severity and incidence of seizures. It has been proven to usefully alleviate the nausea faced by patients undergoing chemotherapy. Marijuana has been touted as a potential substitute for pain management, in place of opioids—powerful painkillers that carry a high risk of addiction. Marijuana has even been considered as a treatment for PTSD, a condition afflicting soldiers and other people who have witnessed traumatic events.

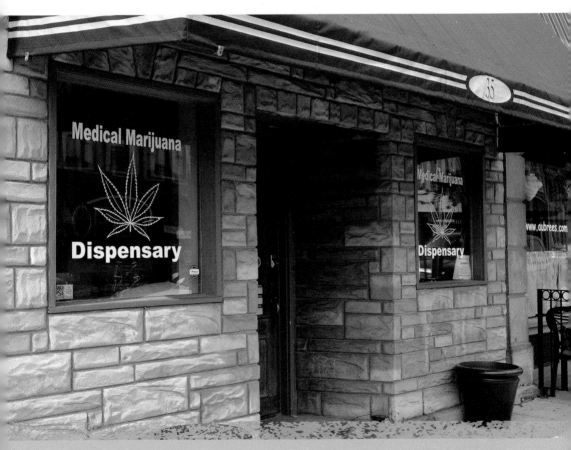

Medical marijuana dispensaries, such as this one in Ypsilanti, Michigan, began opening after the Michigan Medical Marijuana Act was passed in 2008.

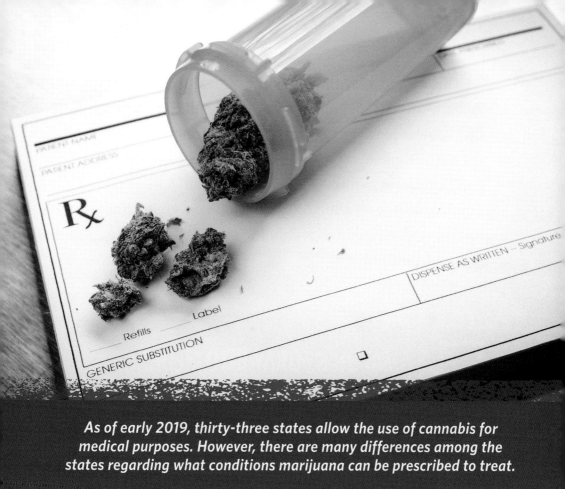

As of early 2019, thirty-three states allow the use of cannabis for medical purposes. However, there are many differences among the states regarding what conditions marijuana can be prescribed to treat.

However, the use of medical marijuana has remained controversial. Although some states have legalized the use of medical marijuana, the federal government continues to classify the drug as having no legitimate medical use, and therefore illegal to possess or consume. Some states that have legalized marijuana for medical purposes have gone on to make recreational use legal as well. This decision is welcomed by civil libertarians, but it has also created a host of headaches for law enforcement and the medical community.

This is not to say that the state of health care in the modern world is all political wrangling and controversy. CIO Review suggests that technological innovation is on the cusp of upending the way we go to the doctor and seek health services in more profound ways than have occurred in many decades. "A majority of consumers are inclined towards these advanced technologies as they have the

AMAZON'S FORAY INTO MEDICINE

According to Knowledge@Wharton, a publication of the Wharton School of Business, Amazon.com is getting into the health care business in a big way. Its latest venture is called Comprehend Medical, a new product by Amazon Web Services that will scan a person's medical records and then use AI and machine learning tools to analyze the data contained within. "Essentially, it is a natural language processing service that pores through medical text for insights into disease conditions, medications and treatment outcomes from patient notes and other electronic health records."[6]

The idea is that the system will empower both doctors and patients to discover new treatments and to lower health care administrative costs. Amazon, potential to transform the health care sector to make it faster and more accessible to the needy."[5]

Some of the innovations involve the way health care providers process information and then use it to devise the best therapies available. A technique called "predictive analytics" will be able to take a patient's past and current medical information and then try to foresee probable outcomes for various therapies. Artificial intelligence will analyze that data and devise solutions faster than human doctors can ever hope to. Block-chain technology will be help keep health care information secure. "In simple

through its tools used to ascertain the preferences of its customers that use its online store, is adept at analyzing seemingly unrelated data and developing useful information from it. Of course, the downside of the new system is the possible threat to patient privacy.

Amazon has also purchased an online pharmacy called Pillpack and is developing a business that will deliver monthly medications to chronically ill patients. The company has also teamed up with Berkshire Hathaway and JP Morgan Chase to devise a health care system that will improve the quality and lower the costs of health care for their employees. If the venture succeeds it might prove to be a useful model for other companies.

terms, a blockchain can be described as an append-only transaction ledger," explains Arthur Linuma in *Forbes*. "What that means is that the ledger can be written onto with new information, but the previous information, stored in blocks, cannot be edited, adjusted or changed."[7] Thus a person's health care information cannot be access or altered by hackers.

One exciting emerging technology is called **telemedicine**, which involves a patient and a doctor interacting over great distances. Using computer interfaces such as Skype, a doctor at a large city hospital could consult with a patient in a rural area without having to be physically present, bringing his or her expertise to people who often live hundreds of miles away from the nearest physician. Telemedicine is also useful for consulting specialists far quicker than the old method of setting up face-to-face appointments.

Robotic surgery does not, despite the name, mean having an autonomous electronic surgeon opening up patients and poking around inside them. Robotic surgery involves a computer-operated device that a human doctor can use to perform surgical procedures with greater precision than ever before, improving outcomes. As the Mayo Clinic explains, "Robotic surgery, or robot-assisted surgery, allows doctors to perform many types of complex procedures with more precision, flexibility and control than is possible with conventional techniques. Robotic surgery is usually associated with minimally invasive surgery—procedures

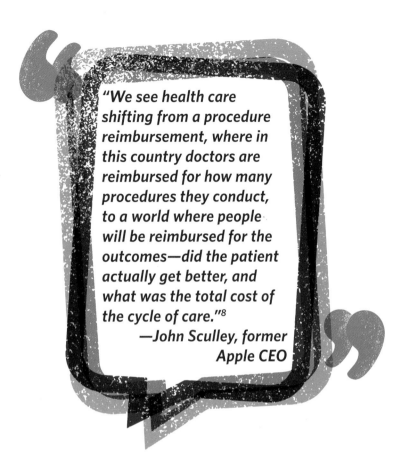

performed through tiny incisions. It is also sometimes used in certain traditional open surgical procedures."[9]

The so-called **internet of things** is related to telemedicine in the sense that it provides medical information to health care professionals instantly and over great distances. The idea is that someone will wear or even have implanted a suite of sensors that will constantly monitor their health. These kinds of sensors can monitor things like heart rate, blood pressure, and so on. Down the road, more sophisticated sensors will be able to detect and relay information such as blood glucose, the interactions of medicine in a human

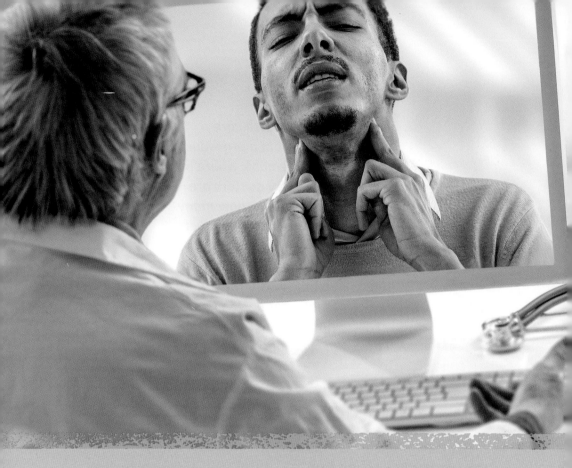

Telemedicine allows doctors to communicate with patients or consult with colleagues over long distances. Studies indicate that telemedicine can reduce the cost of health care, while also improving the quality of care.

body, and even whether or not a person is starting to develop cancer cells. If something amiss is detected, a doctor or other health care provider can alert the patient. A person with medical sensors could even access his or her own data through a wifi network on a computer or smart phone.

Stem cell technology, married sometimes with 3D printing, promises to change the way damaged organs are repaired and even replaced. A heart that has been damaged by a coronary incident can have stem cells implanted, causing the damaged parts to be replaced, making the organ as good as new. Researchers are developing ways to grow entirely new organs using stem cells to be implanted in a patient who needs them.

Totally regrown organs, such as a heart or kidney, would be genetically identical to the ones that are being replaced. When the technology is available, a person in need of a new organ will no longer have to wait for a donor version to become available because it will be grown in a lab from his or her own stem cells. Because the new organ will be genetically identical, a patient will no longer have to take a lifelong regimen of anti-rejection drugs.

The really exciting area of medical research is in the area of lifespan extension. According to a recent piece in *Futurism*, "more and more scientists are coming to the conclusion that aging is a disease and, as such, could be treated."[10] Researchers are developing treatments that can slow or even reverse the aging process. Since human beings tend to get sicker and are prone to more injuries as they age, such treatments will have a profound effect on how we maintain our health.

The concept of "healthspan" concerns not only extending life, but also healthy life. Living to 100 or 120 years would not be very fun if those additional decades were spent as an invalid. However, if good health can be extended along with lifespan, the effects on how people age would be profound indeed. The idea that people have to retire at sixty-five years old or so would become a thing of the past, allowing them to continue their careers or even seek new ones. Death would likely never be abolished, but it could be put off for a long time.

Of course, a lot of technological advances in health care have tradeoffs. New medical technologies can do wondrous things: cure previously incurable diseases, increase well-being, and allow for diseases to be caught early and treated before they become more serious. On the other hand, advances in medicine come with a price. Researchers spend many billions of dollars to develop new drugs and new treatments. Whether the money is paid by the government, private charities, or profit-making companies, it has to have a return.

However, one return on investment can be that a formerly expensive way to deal with a disease can be replaced with an inexpensive cure or even a preventive measure, such as a vaccine. For example, until the mid-1950s people who were infected with the polio virus often had to undergo expensive measures to handle the disease. Children sometimes had to spend their time in a device called an iron lung to help them breathe. People who survived polio often lived the rest of their lives with mobility issues, confined to a wheelchair or forced to get around on crutches. With the advent of the Salk vaccine, a simple injection renders immunity to polio. In the developed world few people contract polio any longer.

Other vaccines have nearly eradicated a host of childhood diseases, such as measles, mumps, and chicken pox. In the past such diseases were just a part of growing up. Most children pulled through, but a few did suffer permanent injuries or even death.

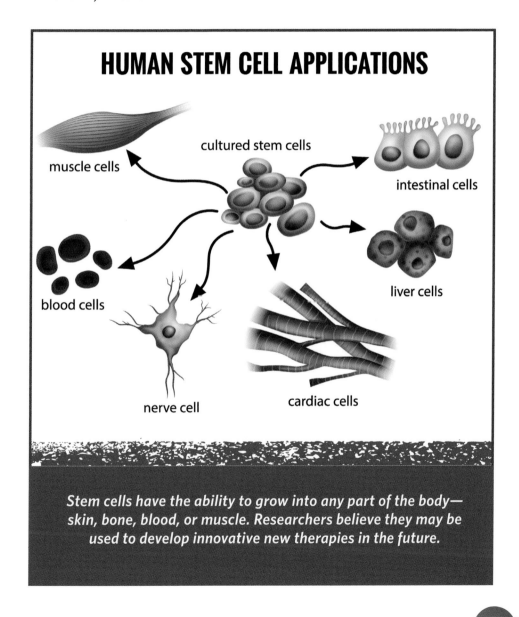

HUMAN STEM CELL APPLICATIONS

muscle cells

cultured stem cells

intestinal cells

blood cells

nerve cell

cardiac cells

liver cells

Stem cells have the ability to grow into any part of the body—skin, bone, blood, or muscle. Researchers believe they may be used to develop innovative new therapies in the future.

Imagine, then, that in the future a simple injection or pill could cure cancer. Researchers are working on medications that would seek and destroy cancer cells like a team of Navy SEALs does enemy targets—with precision and speed. When these new therapies become available, the horror of cancer treatment, with months of chemotherapy accompanied by nausea and pain, could become as much a part of medical history as the iron lung. Not only would many lives be saved, but a great health care expense would have been eliminated. The pharmaceutical industry, which makes billions of dollars on drugs to treat the disease, would be disrupted. Companies will have to adapt and look for future opportunities or die out.

Eliminating once-deadly diseases could cause a great deal of economic chaos. Entire industries have grown up to treat and manage chronic diseases such as cancer and a variety of cardiovascular ailments. If these and other diseases could be treated easily and cheaply, the reason for much of the health care sector might cease to exist. This development could be great for patients, who would live longer, healthier lives, but it might not so good for people employed by companies that profit from expensive treatments for those diseases. However, technological advances inevitably cause this kind of "creative destruction" that ends old industries and creates new ones. Hardly anyone today is selling buggy whips or oxen-pulled plows, after all.

Finally, one of the cutting-edge, almost science-fiction developments involves manipulation of the human genome. Many people have genes that make them more prone to ailments such as cancer and HIV/AIDS. Some genetic abnormalities result in lifelong conditions such as Down syndrome. What if ways were developed to eliminate these genes, to make people while still inside the womb less likely to come down with often fatal diseases? According to the magazine *Science*, a Chinese researcher named Hei Jainkui claims that he has already created genetically modified twins using a tool called CRISPER. He announced that he has created two babies that are now resistant to HIV/AIDS infection. "Hei's goal was to introduce a rare, natural genetic variation that makes it more difficult for HIV to infect its favorite target, white blood cells. Specifically, he deleted a region of a receptor on the surface of white blood cells known as CCR5 using the revolutionary genome-editing technique called CRISPR-Cas9."[11]

Hei's **genetic therapy** experiment is considered controversial because it involves changing genetic material that

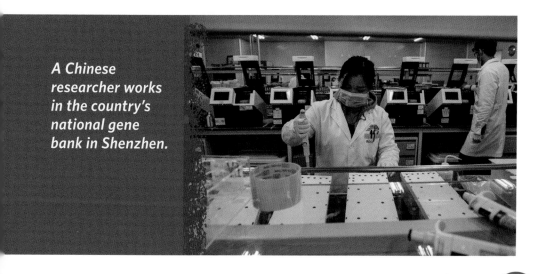

A Chinese researcher works in the country's national gene bank in Shenzhen.

can then be passed along to the infants' potential offspring. Most experiments along these lines involve the alteration of cells that are not passed along, with the goal of curing such diseases as muscular dystrophy and sickle-cell anemia. Hei seems to have created human beings who will pass along the traits he engineered to their offspring.

Naturally, Hei's announcement has touched off a debate about how far scientists should go in changing the human genome. Besides some scientists' belief that such experiments are, at best, premature, ethical questions are being asked about the technique. The benefits of eliminating disease would seem to be a no-brainer. But what if people decided to create what would be in effect, "super babies?" Such children would have enhanced intelligence, athletic ability, even better creativity. They would tend to live longer than ordinary people. Would human beings take evolution into their control and start creating the successors to homo sapiens? What would happen to ordinary, non-enhanced people in a world in which such enhanced humans are possible? Will such treatments be available to everyone or just to people who can afford it?

In short, while public policy questions continue to bedevil health care, advances in technology have the potential for a bright future in which many diseases become things of the past. The challenge to make sound choices remains, however. In other words, developing cures for diseases is easy. Making sure that those cures are available to everyone is hard.

TEXT-DEPENDENT QUESTIONS

1. What was a positive result of the Affordable Care Act?
2. What is telemedicine?
3. What is robotic surgery?

 RESEARCH PROJECTS

Write a two-page paper proposing a new health care system for the United States. You can borrow some of the ideas being advanced by politicians and public policy experts, but do not be afraid to be creative and come up with your own solutions. Explain how your new system would deliver the best quality health care at the lowest cost for the most people.

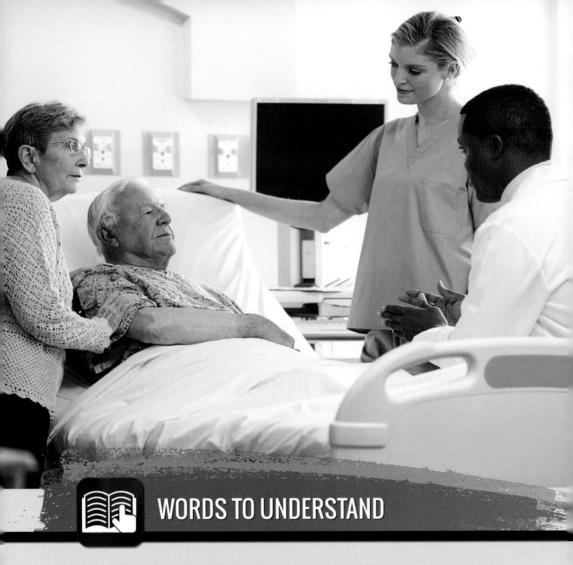

WORDS TO UNDERSTAND

catastrophic health insurance—a health care policy with a high deductible but with low premiums. It is designed to cover the costs of expensive long-term conditions such as cancer or injuries resulting from a severe accident.

National Health Service—government-run health care in the United Kingdom.

universal health care—a term used to describe proposals for a single government-run health care system that would be provided to everyone in the United States. Such programs are also known as "single-payer" or "Medicare for all."

WOULD UNIVERSAL SINGLE-PAYER HEALTH CARE BE EFFECTIVE?

CHAPTER 2

The concept of health care as a human right has gained a great deal of popularity in recent years. The idea is that no one should go without medical attention simply because of an inability to pay for the service. But how does a government guarantee this right? Most rights, such as the ones of free speech or to keep and bear arms, involve the government being forbidden to stop people from doing things. The right to free health care involves the government giving citizens something with a tangible cost.

The concept of the government providing health care has been touted as a solution to the question of how to grant the service as a right. Whether the concept is called **universal health care**, single-payer health care, or even, as Senator Bernie Sanders terms it, "Medicare for all," the system would involve the government levying a tax to pay for the service and establishing a government-run (or at least government-funded) system of doctors and hospitals. People would be able to see the doctor or go to the hospital without having to worry about paying the cost of their care, at least directly.

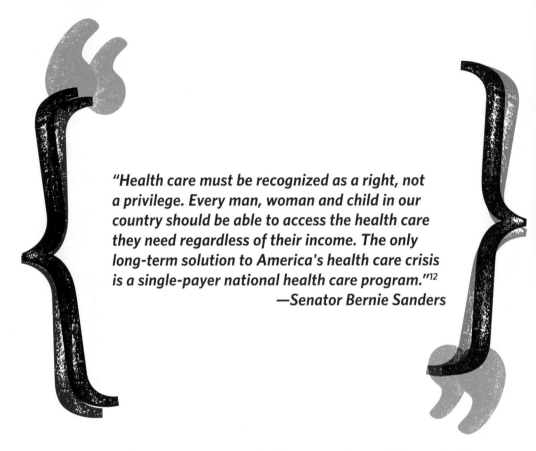

"Health care must be recognized as a right, not a privilege. Every man, woman and child in our country should be able to access the health care they need regardless of their income. The only long-term solution to America's health care crisis is a single-payer national health care program."[12]
—*Senator Bernie Sanders*

Many other countries, including Canada and the United Kingdom, have a form of universal health care. Even the United States provides health care for specific populations. For example, Medicare is a health insurance program for elderly and disabled Americans. Poor Americans are eligible for a similar program, called Medicaid. Military veterans are often eligible for treatment through the health system run by the Veterans Administration (VA), especially when medical conditions are related to injuries incurred during their military service.

Still, the arguments for and against a government-run or funded health care system continue to rage in the United States.

UNIVERSAL HEALTH CARE WOULD BE EFFECTIVE

Proponents of a universal health care system that is provided by the government point out that the cost of medical treatments is skyrocketing. Medical science has developed therapies that would have been considered miraculous a generation ago. However, those treatments come with a high cost. Only a government, with its vast resources, is capable of getting a handle on those costs and making these life-saving treatments available to all citizens.

The arguments supporting a government-run universal health care system in the United States can be divided into two categories: "moral" and "economic."

In the moral column, a study by the American Medical Student Association (AMSA) suggests that under a program of universal health care, people would no longer worry that medical costs would be unaffordable. People who need the services of a doctor will just go and get treatment without worrying about how to pay for it. Such a system would therefore take away a lot of the psychological stress that health care causes. If one gets sick, one gets treatment.

"At its root, the lack of health care for all in America is fundamentally a moral issue," note the AMSA study's authors. "The United States is the only industrialized nation that does not have some form of universal health care (defined as a basic guarantee of health care to all of its citizens). While other countries have declared health care to be a basic right, the United States treats health care as a privilege, only available to those who can afford it. In this sense, health care in America is treated as an economic good like a TV or VCR, not as a social or public good."[13]

An egalitarian aspect exists for universal health care. Under the current system, the well-to-do have access to some of the beat health care on the planet. However, even the middle class with health insurance, not to mention the poor with no insurance, are faced with deductibles and copays that can eat up even an upper-middle-class income fairly quickly if an expensive disease such as cancer presents itself. Under universal health care, everybody gets treated, regardless of their wealth or income.

The economic and health costs of a lack of universal health care can be enormous. People without insurance are more likely to delay seeking health care services, not fill their prescriptions, and thus suffer more from chronic diseases. People without insurance are more likely to die from treatable diseases such as cancer, AIDS, or cardiovascular ailments. The psychological stress of going without insurance can be profound, as well. Stress can exacerbate the physical effects of untreated illness.

The economic effects of an expensive disease can also be profound, even for those people with health insurance. Those effects include a higher rate of bankruptcy, lost wages, and the necessity of cutting back on other spending to pay for out-of-pocket health care costs. Under a universal health care system, those economic effects would be alleviated. People would no longer have to choose between paying out-of-pocket health care costs and, say, food or

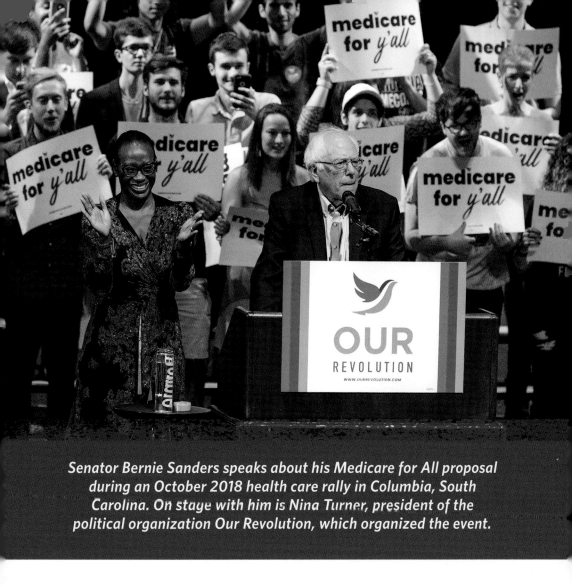

Senator Bernie Sanders speaks about his Medicare for All proposal during an October 2018 health care rally in Columbia, South Carolina. On stage with him is Nina Turner, president of the political organization Our Revolution, which organized the event.

housing. They would not have to resort to setting up a GoFundMe campaign to literally beg for money to pay such costs. A great deal of worry and stress associated with being sick would not exist.

The AMSA article also presents a number of economic arguments in support of universal health care. The core of the analysis delves into the question of whether the cost of initiating such a system would be balanced by its economic benefits. The short answer is, yes.

The report claims that the costs of creating a universal health care system is about $34 to 64 billion a year, plus "whatever costs are associated with covering out-of-pocket expenses and uncompensated care for the uninsured."[14]

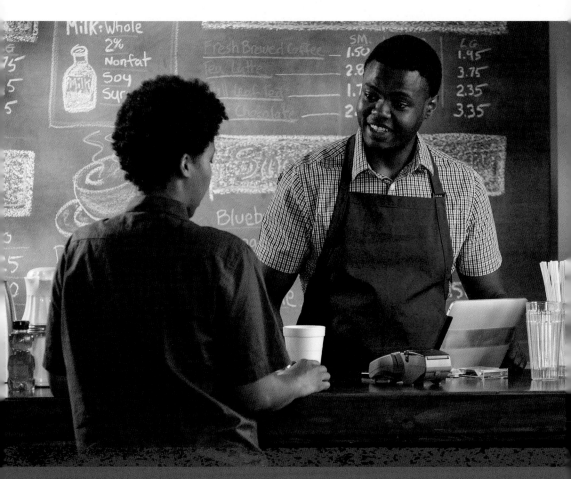

Many stores and restaurants do not offer health benefits to their employees. For a worker who is making a low hourly wage, purchasing a health insurance plan can be prohibitively expensive.

The piece also suggests that there will be some additional, unspecified costs as well, but nothing that cannot be borne by a rich country such as the United States.

However, the article claims that the savings from a universal health care system would more than pay for the costs of creating it. People would be healthier through greater access to health care. This would enable them to work longer and have more earning power. With health care for all, children would be able to develop at a faster pace, enhancing their ability to became educated and join the work force.

Both businesses and workers would benefit from a universal government-provided health care system, Businesses would no longer have to provide expensive health benefits to their employees, allowing them to reduce operating costs. Companies would have access to a healthier work force, which could improve their productivity. These things would help American businesses to better compete in the global economy. At the same time, workers would be empowered to leave jobs that they did not like, without having to worry that they would lose their health insurance coverage. Workers could use their leverage to demand higher wages and better working conditions, and employers would be better positioned to grant such demands through the savings of not paying employee health benefits.

Taxpayers would also benefit from a universal health care system. Currently, elderly, disabled, and poor Americans receive medical care through Medicare and/

or Medicaid, which are both taxpayer-funded government programs. The costs of those programs could be expected to decrease because Americans in general would be healthier with access to better health care. Medicare and Medicaid could be blended into the larger health care system, providing an opportunity for greater efficiency thanks to the purchasing power of the federal government. A government-run health care system would be better able to negotiate prices with drug companies and medical providers. Drug costs could be subsidized in certain cases to make them more affordable. Additionally, universal health care would eliminate the need for people to access hospital emergency rooms as their primary source of care. This would save the hospitals millions in unpaid expenses, and free the facilities to deal with actual medical emergencies, as they are intended.

Scan here to learn more about how a single-payer system differs from the current health care system.

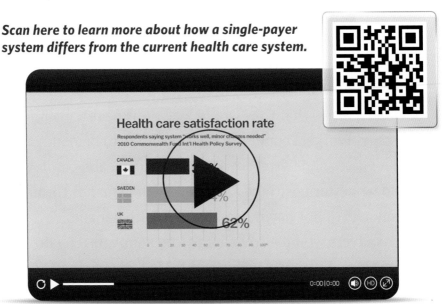

UNIVERSAL HEALTH CARE WOULD NOT BE EFFECTIVE

Universal health care would greatly increase the size of the federal government, while also forcing people off their private health insurance—whether they want to be or not. A universal health care system would likely be a "one-size-fits-all" structure, with little or no freedom of choice. Imposing such a system would be cumbersome at best for a country of over 325 million people. The bureaucracy needed to run and maintain such a system would be mind-numbingly complex, with a decision-making process that would be slow and inflexible.

A major criticism against various schemes to enact a universal health care in the United States has been its cost. The Mercatus Center at George Mason University recently examined the so-called Medicare for All plan proposed by Senator Bernie Sanders. It found that the cost of implementing it over ten years would be $32.6 trillion. This cost is actually conservative, since it takes into account claims by Sanders and his supporters that the plan would reduce drug prices and administrative costs for health care.

The tax increases necessary to pay for a Medicare for All program are likely to be both politically and economically unsustainable. "The federal government would become responsible for financing nearly all current national health spending, including individual private insurance and state spending," writes study author Charles Blahous. "A doubling of all currently projected federal individual and corporate income tax collections would be insufficient to finance the added federal costs of the plan."[15]

With health care spending taking up so much of government resources, less money would be available for other national priorities such as defense and infrastructure. Indeed, the projected costs of universal health care have stopped efforts to enact it on the state level in both Sanders's home state of Vermont and in California, both progressive states where the concept has proven to be popular, at least among the political class.

"With regard to the idea whether or not you have a right to health care you have to realize what that implies. I am a physician. You have a right to come to my house and conscript me. It means you believe in slavery. You are going to enslave not only me but the janitor at my hospital, the person who cleans my office, the assistants, the nurses....You are basically saying you believe in slavery."[16]
—*US Senator Rand Paul, a medical doctor.*

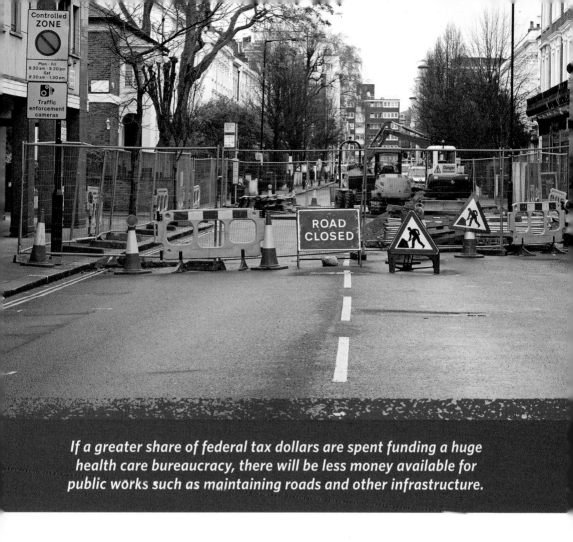

If a greater share of federal tax dollars are spent funding a huge health care bureaucracy, there will be less money available for public works such as maintaining roads and other infrastructure.

Another argument against universal health care stems from how such systems function in practice in other countries. One of those countries is Canada, which has a government-run health care system. A recent report by the Fraser Institute suggests that Canadians spend more on health care, and receive less coverage, than citizens of other countries that have universal health care.[17] Another report from Fraser notes that Canadians endure enormous wait times for medical procedures because

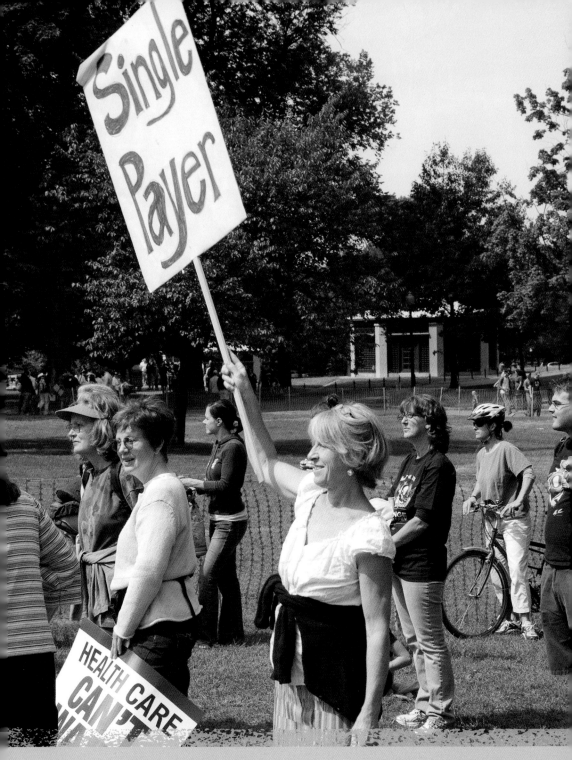

Protesters rally on the Boston Common to support health care reform.

of a lack of health care resources   an average of more than twenty-one weeks between a referral from a general practitioner and the treatment being ordered. The wait times result in pain, suffering, and mental anguish for patients.[18]

The need to wait for treatment sometimes results in poorer medical outcomes, permanent disabilities, and injuries. The loss of wages while waiting for treatment exacts an economic cost on Canadians. In effect, besides taxes, Canadians pay for their "free" health care through the rationing of services and lack of access to the most modern treatments.

What about the British **National Health Service**, another example of universal health care? According to the respected medical journal *The Lancet*, the NHS is also bedeviled with a disconnect between resources and need. NHS doctors face "chronic understaffing, lack of cover, a paucity of senior doctors, long hours, stress, and junior doctors left in charge of large caseloads."[19] While the British people still support their government health care system, clearly some kind of overhaul is needed.

One of the central bodies of the British health care system is the National Institute for Health and Care Excellence (NICE), According to a report by the National Center for Biotechnology Information, NICE acts as a rationing body, determining what medical services will be made available and which ones will be withheld on what it calls a cost/benefit basis. The practical effect is that treatments that may be available outside of the NHS system are being denied to British patients within that system.[20]

One egregious example of health care rationing in the UK was the Liverpool Care Pathway for the Dying Patient (LCP). In theory the LCP was a way to help terminal patients die with a modicum of dignity. In practice, due to economic incentives provided to hospitals, patients were heavily sedated and denied water and nutrients, making

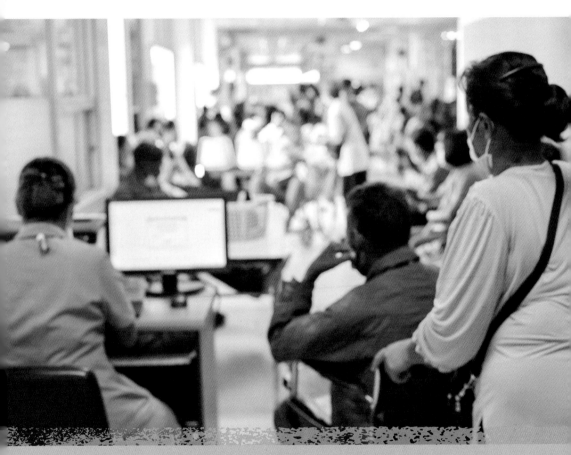

In countries like Canada and the United Kingdom, patients have complained about long wait times for care, and lack of access to certain treatments that the government refuses to provide.

Contemporary Issues: Health Care

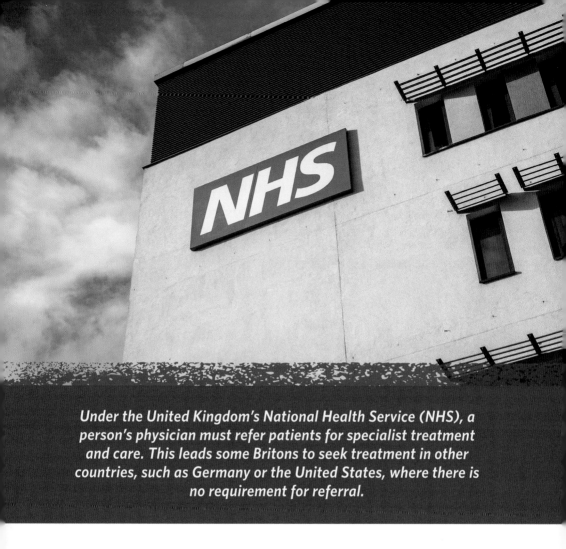

Under the United Kingdom's National Health Service (NHS), a person's physician must refer patients for specialist treatment and care. This leads some Britons to seek treatment in other countries, such as Germany or the United States, where there is no requirement for referral.

the terminal diagnoses self-fulfilling. The system was less about helping patients than it was about helping the NHS save money.[21] The program was discontinued after a media firestorm.

One of the more gut-wrenching examples of how dysfunctional the NHS has become concerns the case of Charlie Gard, a British infant who was diagnosed with a terminal genetic defect. His parents wanted to take their child to the United States for experimental treatment. Even though they had raised the money through a GoFundMe campaign, Charlie's doctors prevented the transfer, citing that it would not be in his best interests to receive treatment. Whether the experimental therapy would have worked is unknown, because Charlie died from his condition because the National Health Service and the courts blocked his parents from trying the treatment. The case remains controversial to this day, pitting the American

WHAT IS MEDI-SHARE?

Medi-Share is a faith-based organization that presents itself as an alternative to individual health insurance. Members contribute a fixed amount of money to an account. When a member needs help paying a medical bill, he or she files a request for reimbursement and, if the request is approved, Medi-Share pays the health care provider for the service rendered.

Organizations like Medi-Share have certain advantages over traditional insurance plans. No lifetime or annual limits on coverage are imposed. Coverage is not dependent on residence or employment. Adoption and funeral expenses are covered as well as health care.

patient-centered health system against the British doctor-centered approach.

The Liverpool Care Pathway scandal and the Charlie Gard story strongly suggest that a universal health care system would remove freedom of choice for patients as to whether they live or die. Cost considerations would inevitably drive such a system to eschew heroic measures to save life, whether they would be successful or not. The right to life is fundamental in any free society. Universal health care, in practice, may well take that right away and place such decisions in the hands of medical bureaucrats. Former Alaska governor and vice presidential candidate

On the other hand, because Medi-Share is a faith-based organization, it imposes strict behavior guidelines on its members. Members must be believing Christians who promise to abstain from tobacco or illegal drugs and to attend church regularly. Certain restrictions and surcharges are imposed for those with preexisting conditions, such a diabetes.

Still, the idea of relatively small groups that share medical expenses may become a viable alternative to both traditional private insurance and government-run universal health care in the next decade.

Sarah Palin was roundly ridiculed when she claimed that the Patient Protection and Affordable Care Act would create "death panels." However, the history of the National Health Service suggests that Palin and other ACA critics had a valid point.

Rather than creating an expensive new health care system, the present system could be improved through free-market reforms. One idea, proposed in the mid-1990s by Andrew Ferris and Griffin Seiler in the Loyola Consumer Law Review, would consist of **catastrophic health care insurance** coupled with medical savings accounts. The funding would be provided by payroll deductions for employees, pretax expenditures for the self-employed, or by the government through Medicare or Medicaid. People would be free to purchase health maintenance insurance with their MSA money or purchase services directly. In theory, patients would shop around for the best and most cost-effective health care services, forcing providers to compete and to be more transparent about their costs and outcomes. Unlike government-run universal health care, the state would not heavily regulate the health care system, mandating treatments and so on as has been the case under the Affordable Care Act. If something like this were implemented, it might work better to provide people with health care services at a cost they can afford.

TEXT-DEPENDENT QUESTIONS

1. What is the estimated cost to implement Senator Bernie Sanders's Medicare for All plan over a ten-year period?

2. What was the purpose of the Liverpool Care Pathway for the Dying Patient? Why did it go wrong?

3. How could the savings from a universal health care system offset the costs of creating such as system?

 RESEARCH PROJECTS

The idea of a government-run and funded universal health care system remains a controversial one. Investigate the plans for bringing about such a program offered by politicians such as Sen. Bernie Sanders and the arguments in favor and against it offered by various politicians and experts.

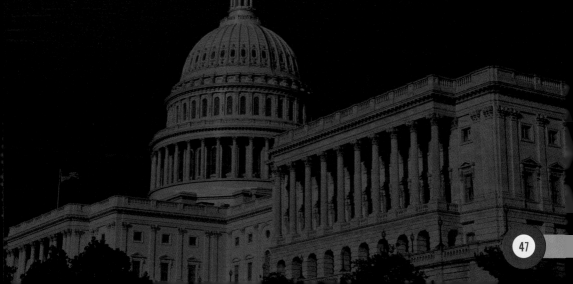

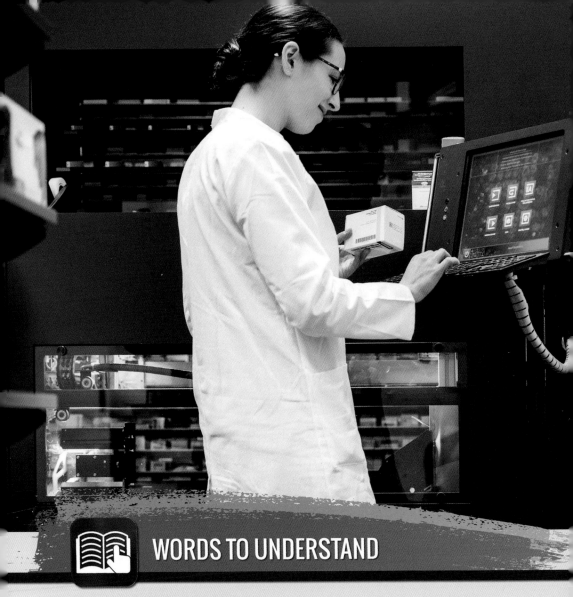

WORDS TO UNDERSTAND

price control—a policy of the government that sets prices for a product, either by direct edict or by indirect means.

monopoly—a situation in which only one company produces a particular product or offers a particular service.

SHOULD THE COST OF DRUGS BE SUBJECT TO PRICE CONTROLS?

CHAPTER 3

Americans of every political persuasion agree that drug prices have become too expensive and are increasing at a dizzying rate. According to a study by the US Bureau of Labor Statistics, prices for prescription drugs were 85 percent higher in 2018 than they were in 2000. During that period, the rate of inflation increased by 2.12 percent. The figure does not account for price increases for life-saving equipment such as epi-pens and drugs like insulin, which have ballooned many times over in recent years.

The sticking point is not only why these price increases are taking place, but what to do about it.

Because high drug prices can often mean life or death for people who need them, the question has generated a lot of heat in the media. However, the National Center for Biotechnology Information has a stark reason for drug price inflation: "The noise level in the news regarding drug prices (eg, EpiPen, generics) has been high. So who's to blame? How about everyone! It is easy to point the finger at a few greedy people and the pharmaceutical industry, but the whole system is the problem. This includes patients, the insurance industry, employers, legislators, the boards of

directors of pharmaceutical companies, CEOs of pharmaceutical companies, and the stockholders of any company
associated with the production and pricing of the pharmaceuticals. Each of these has contributed to the problem and
is negatively affected, directly and indirectly."[22]

Patients don't necessarily notice the higher cost of
medications when they are covered by government health
care programs, such as Medicare and Medicaid, or by
private insurance. However, insurance companies or the
government have to adapt to the increasing cost of drugs.
Often, the cost increases are offset either by higher premiums, or by reductions in coverage.

A recent Harvard Medical School study suggested that
high drug prices are primarily the result of well-inten-
tioned government policies. "The 'most important factor'
that drives prescription drug prices higher in the United
States than anywhere else in the world is the existence of
government-protected **monopoly** rights for drug manufacturers," noted the report.[23]

Unlike elsewhere in the world, drug companies can
set their own prices in the United States. While Medicaid
is allowed to get a discount for medications, Medicare is
not allowed to negotiate drug prices with pharmaceutical
companies.

In order to foster innovation, the government allows
drug companies to be the sole proprietor of drugs they
develop for as long as twenty years before generic versions
are allowed on the market. Some drug companies use

sneaky methods to maintain what is in effect a monopoly by tweaking the characteristics of their drugs and paying off potential manufacturers of generics to wait before releasing cheaper versions. The Food and Drug Administration is also tardy in approving new generic versions of existing drugs. And some state and local laws require medical professionals to gain a patients' consent before switching them from a brand-name drug to a generic drug.

The Harvard Medical School study also disputes the often-cited reason for high drug costs, that being the cost of research and development. The study notes that the development of new drugs is often funded by government grants to academic labs, or by private capital.

When a monopoly exists, with only a single drug to treat a disease, companies will often charge whatever they

To learn more about why US drug prices are so high, scan here.

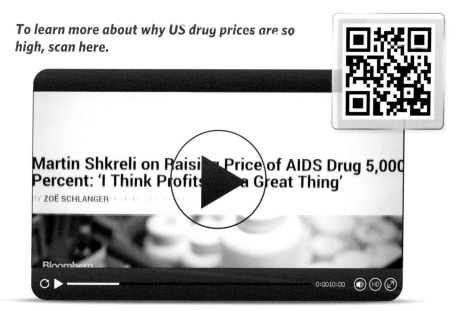

Martin Shkreli on Raising Price of AIDS Drug 5,000 Percent: 'I Think Profits a Great Thing'

BY ZOË SCHLANGER

Bloomberg

0:00 | 0:00

think the market will bear. The problem is that, in some cases, patients can't bear the price increases.

According to the American Medical Association, there are three major players who determine the price of drugs in America. Pharmaceutical companies make and sell drugs intending to make a profit. Pharmacy benefit managers (PBMs) work on behalf of health insurance companies or employers to negotiate upfront discounts on the prices of prescription drugs with pharmaceutical companies, as well as rebates, which reward the insurance companies for increasing the use of a particular drug by its patients. These prescription drug agreements are kept secret, so it is unknown if savings ever reach the patients. And the health insurance companies themselves approve treatments, establish co-pays, and price out with pharmacy benefit managers how much patients pay for drugs. Often, they select the coverage options that will maximize company profits.

The factors governing the price of drugs in America are complicated and often opaque, which encourages high drug prices. So how can the high cost of drugs be reduced? Is the solution just as complicated as the problem? Or can something simple be done to cut through the complexity to solve the problem?

STRICT PRICE CONTROLS ON DRUGS ARE NEEDED

Virtually every argument for slapping **price controls** on drugs starts with a moral dimension. No one should have to die or suffer from a chronic disease just because they cannot afford the drugs that would save their lives or alleviate the symptoms of their disease. The very idea of such a thing happening in a wealthy country such as the United States offends the conscience. The argument that price controls would be a good way to address the problem of drug price inflation in the United States also points to the success that policy has enjoyed in other countries.

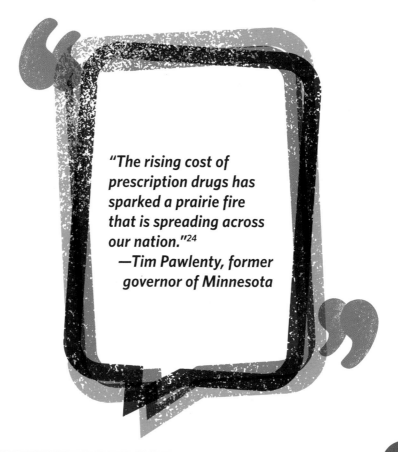

"The rising cost of prescription drugs has sparked a prairie fire that is spreading across our nation."[24]
—Tim Pawlenty, former governor of Minnesota

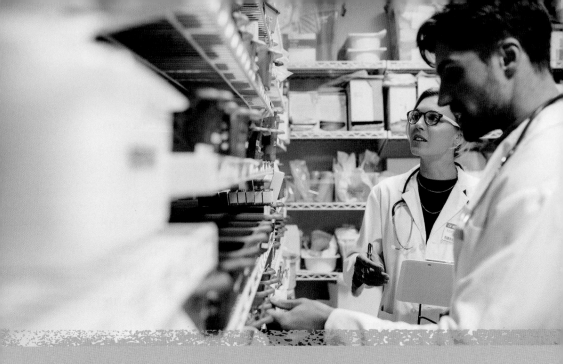

Drugs in the United States are between three and six times more expensive than they are in other countries. High drug costs are a key element of increasing health care costs in general.

Such is the stance taken by an article in the *Harvard Political Review*, "To promote public health and ensure that patients are able to fulfill their prescriptions at a reasonable price, American policymakers thus have a moral obligation to replicate the success that other countries have already had in instituting price controls on drugs," writes analyst Michael Wornow.[25]

His essay also offers some economic arguments for implementing drug price controls.

"Despite accounting for over 40 percent of global spending on prescription drugs, American patients may still be falling short of their recommended dosages," notes

Wornow. "According to a study published in the *Annals of Internal Medicine*, roughly 30 percent of all pharmaceutical prescriptions in the United States are 'never filled,' which has directly led to almost $300 billion in avoidable health care costs annually and roughly 125,000 deaths from patients failing to adhere to their prescriptions. This would be the sixth leading cause of death in America. Accordingly, the World Health Organization has written that increasing adherence to prescriptions would have a 'far greater impact on the health of the population than any improvement in specific medical treatments.'"[26]

In fact, in a recent National Public Radio poll, 67 percent of respondents cited the high cost of medications as a reason for not filling their prescriptions. The figure is 95 percent for respondents who reported incomes under $25,000 a year.

Price caps on expensive, name-brand drugs would increase the number of patients who fill their prescriptions and therefore take the medications. That conclusion is Economics 101. The less anything costs, the more people will be inclined to buy it. In the case of drugs, lowering the price means that more people will live, and more people who do live will be healthy.

According to Wornow, price caps on drugs would increase their usage by patients, and would barely affect pharmaceutical company profits—possibly lowering them by as little as 1 percent. Contrary to the claims of the companies, drug innovation would not be impacted adversely.

The article does not mention the indirect effects of more people being alive and healthy because of better access to drugs, but it bears mentioning. These people would be able to work, start businesses, and otherwise be productive, adding value to the economy, rather than being mourned by their friends and relatives.

How would a system of drug price controls work in the United States? Other countries, such as Canada and Great Britain, have some form of universal, government health care, enhancing their ability to set drug prices.

Canada has a complex system in which both the federal government and the provincial governments have input into how much medications cost. According to Health Affairs, "Governments in Canada have instituted mechanisms intended to control drug prices. These include the establishment of a semi-judicial body by the federal government to control factory-gate prices and of various measures at the provincial level, such as formulary management, use of generics, reference-based pricing, price freezes, and limits on markups. To a large extent, these measures have been effective in price control."[27]

Great Britain employs a strict cost/benefit analysis to determine the price and availability of drugs. "A voluntary system called the Pharmaceutical Price Regulation Scheme (PPRS) is the primary touchstone for setting drug prices in the UK," notes an article in *Pharmaceutical Technology*. "The PPRS is a non-contractual agreement between the UK Department of Health and the members of the Association of the British Pharmaceutical Industry (ABPI), and is usually reviewed every five years. The current iteration ... uses a value-based pricing mechanism and limits the profits that pharma companies can make from drug sales to the NHS, rather than the prices themselves."[28]

Unless the United States were to switch from the combination of government health care (Medicare, Medicaid, etc.) and private insurance, it would have to find another mechanism to cap drug prices. The Food and Drug Administration approves the availability of drugs in the American market. The determination of price caps could certainly be added to the FDA's mandate. The government could then set prices based on equivalent prices in foreign markets, how much out-of-pocket expense the private company bore in developing the drug, how urgent the need is for the particular drug, and other factors. The NIH could increase spending on new drug research, lowering the cost that would have to be borne by individual patients.

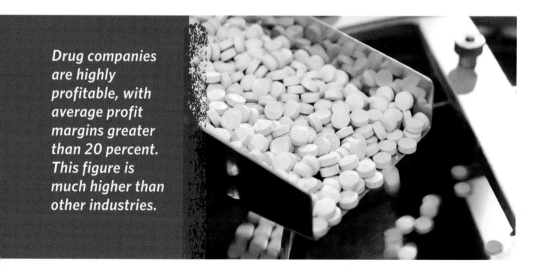

Drug companies are highly profitable, with average profit margins greater than 20 percent. This figure is much higher than other industries.

STRICT PRICE CONTROLS ON DRUGS ARE NOT NEEDED

The main argument against imposing strict price controls on drugs is the belief by many free-market economists that price controls do not work in the long run. Wayne Winegarden, Ph.D., a senior fellow in business and economics at the Pacific Research Institute, policy advisor to the Heartland Institute, and the managing editor for *EconoSTATS*, suggested in a recent *Forbes* essay that the problem with high drug prices is systematic within the health care system.

"For instance, the health care system unnecessarily obstructs competition in the practice of medicine and has failed to effectively embrace the information technology revolution. Other policies, such as the inefficiencies inherent in our current health care payment model or the excessive costs created by the tort liability system, are currently dis-incenting innovations and best practices. Fundamental reforms in these areas will meaningfully reduce health care costs while improving overall health care quality."[29]

Information technology would be the key to bringing transparency to drug prices and fostering competition. Winegarden also suggests that tort reform, limiting the amount of money that can be awarded in medical malpractice suits, will contribute to lowering both drug prices and health care costs in general.

Arguing against price controls for drugs, Citizens Against Government Waste suggests that they have always caused shortages, citing examples ranging from attempts at fixing prices at the Massachusetts Bay Colony in the 1630s to the wage and price controls enacted in the 1970s during the Nixon Administration. Attempts to fix prices have also caused producers to get creative to evade the law. Price controls for drugs simply would not work, in the view of the GACW, even if it were tried indirectly through rebates.

"The best way to lower consumer prices for pharmaceuticals is to encourage a vibrant, competitive marketplace, not overlay more government intervention in drug pric-

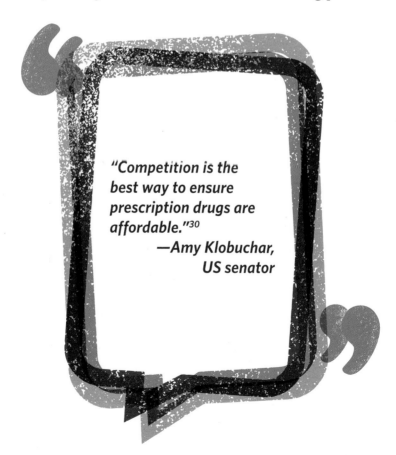

"Competition is the best way to ensure prescription drugs are affordable."[30]
—Amy Klobuchar, US senator

ing," suggests a Citizens Against Government Waste press release. "Using modern scientific methods and improving performance at the FDA would enable research-based and generic pharmaceuticals to enter the marketplace faster."[31]

It takes about ten to twelve years to complete all of

 ## WHY ARE INSULIN PRICES SO HIGH?

By every economic law, insulin prices should not be as high as they are now. Insulin is not a new drug, as it has been around since the 1920s. Three companies make insulin, which people with type 1 diabetes must take on a regular basis in order to live.

Yet, the media is filled with horror stories of people with diabetes who are confronted with prices of as much as $1,300 for a month's supply. Some lower-income patients have taken the dangerous approach of rationing their insulin intake, risking an early death. How did this happen?

GoodRX, a website and mobile app that tracks drug prices, notes that a new form of insulin, called analog insulin, was developed in the 1990s. It is more effective than older forms (human insulin), but also more expensive to manufacture. Also, because the analog version is a "biologic," using bacteria and recombinant DNA technology in its manufacture, FDA regulations the clinical trials necessary to get the FDA to approve a new drug. Some drugs in development do not pan out for various reasons. User fees have funded the FDA approval process, speeding it up in certain cases. More should be done to speed the approval process for new drugs and new versions of drugs, the better to create a vibrant, competitive marketplace. Thus, with more choices and more competition, the price of drugs will start decreasing and not continue increasing. Recently, the price of Sovaldi, a

for approving generic versions are more stringent.

Moreover, the three insulin manufacturers—Sanofi, Eli Lilly, and Novo Nordisk—have been hit by a class action lawsuit claiming a price-fixing scheme. Insulin prices are set artificially high, but then are sold at a huge discount. Unfortunately the discount is not often passed along to patients. High-deductible copay insurance policies also contribute to the problem.

GoodRx suggests a number of strategies for avoiding high insulin prices, including switching to older, synthetic versions of human insulin that some studies suggest are just as good at controlling blood sugar as the newer analog kind. "Due to the added convenience and benefits of analog insulin, 96 percent of insulin prescriptions in the U.S. are now for analogs," notes medical writer Marie Beaugureau. "However, a growing body of research suggests that synthetic human insulin is just as effective for managing diabetes."[32]

hepatitis C drug, increased by its manufacturer Gilead to $84,000 for a 12-week course. When other drug companies rolled out their own hepatitis C drugs, Sovaldi's price dropped.

Expensive drugs also tend to offset other medical procedures that are even more expensive. "Unfortunately, there is little discussion about the other side of the ledger: how much the hepatitis C drugs save in future medical costs by curing people of a chronic disease and keeping them out of the hospital, making liver transplants unnecessary, and allowing patients to become productive citizens."[33] Even an expensive drug can reduce overall health care cost if it replaces a surgical procedure.

To sum up the argument against price controls, the key to lowering and limiting the price of drugs, in the view of those who oppose price controls, is transparency concerning price and effectiveness, combined with a free market with lots of choices and competition. Such a system will discourage drug manufacturers from taking advantage of their government-sanctioned monopolies on certain medications by raising their price to stratospheric levels. Competitors would have an incentive to develop similar drugs to treat the same illness, causing price competition.

TEXT-DEPENDENT QUESTIONS

1. What three entities are responsible for the high price of drugs?
2. When are generic versions of drugs allowed on the market?
3. What is the role of pharmacy benefit managers in determining drug prices?

 RESEARCH PROJECTS

Find a list of drugs similar to insulin that are used to manage chronic diseases. Use Google to research what cures for these diseases are undergoing clinical trials. The idea is to ascertain how expensive drugs can be replaced with a once-and-for-all cure. An historic example is how the polio vaccine eliminated the need to manage polio, including the use of devices such as the iron lung.

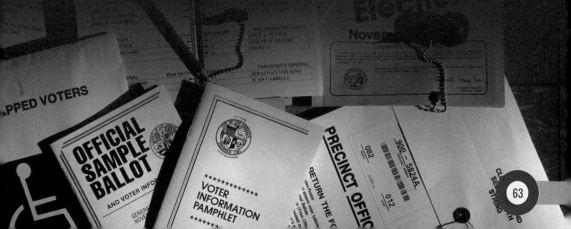

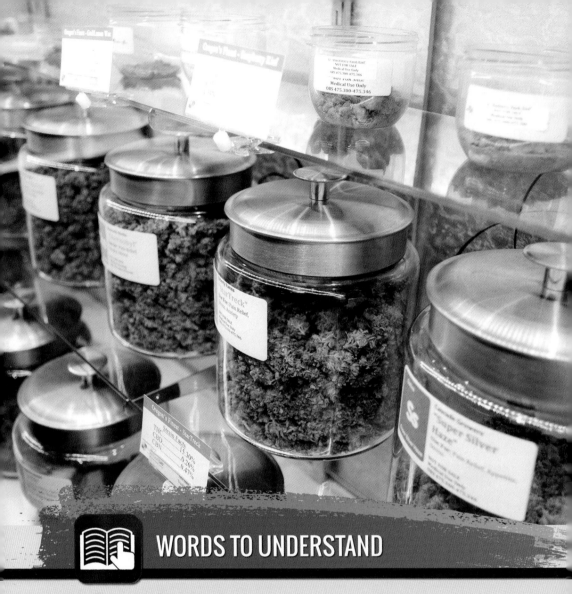

WORDS TO UNDERSTAND

cholera—an infectious bacterial disease of the small intestine that causes severe vomiting and diarrhea. It was often fatal until drugs were developed to treat the infection.

psychoactive—the effect of a drug on the brain and central nervous system, which results in temporary changes to mood, perception, consciousness, and behavior.

recreational marijuana—cannabis that is smoked or ingested for the pleasurable "high" it delivers, rather than for any medical purpose.

SHOULD ALL STATES APPROVE MEDICAL MARIJUANA?

CHAPTER 4

The plant *Cannabis sativa*—commonly known as marijuana—has been used for medicinal purposes since ancient times. Because of its **psychoactive** effect, which users refer to as a "high," it is also a popular recreational drug. Use of cannabis may have started in Asia about 500 BCE, eventually spreading into Europe and the rest of the world. The Greek writer Herodotus noted that the Scythians, a nomadic people who lived in central Asia, used a form of cannabis for both recreational and religious purposes.

Cannabis was introduced to western medicine during the nineteenth century. In the 1830s, Sir William Brooke O'Shaughnessy, an Irish doctor who was studying in India, found that cannabis extracts could help reduce stomach cramps and vomiting in people suffering from **cholera**. By the late 1800s, cannabis extracts were sold in pharmacies and doctors' offices throughout Europe and the United States to treat stomach problems and other ailments.

Scientists later discovered that THC—the compound that causes marijuana's mind-altering effects—was also responsible for marijuana's medicinal properties. THC

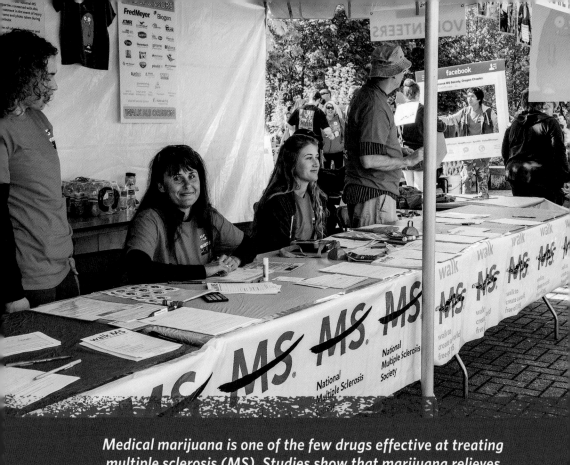

Medical marijuana is one of the few drugs effective at treating multiple sclerosis (MS). Studies show that marijuana relieves muscle stiffness and other symptoms of MS.

interacts with areas of the brain that lessen nausea and promote hunger.

During the 1930s, marijuana use for either **recreational** or medicinal purposes was outlawed in the United States. In 1970, a federal law called the Controlled Substance Act created five classifications of drugs, called "schedules." Marijuana was placed on Schedule 1, meaning that it has a high probability of abuse and no legitimate medicinal use. Despite being illegal, marijuana remained a popular recreational drug, especially among young people.

Over the next few decades, some medical researchers worked to show that cannabis did in fact have legitimate medicinal uses, and should be removed from Schedule 1. By 1996, marijuana's medicinal uses were recognized enough that California became the first state to legalize its use for limited purposes to manage chronic medical conditions. Today the use of medical marijuana is legal in thirty-three states, the District of Columbia, and Puerto Rico. Some of these states have also legalized marijuana for recreational use, albeit in a heavily regulated setting. Despite this, marijuana remains on the federal Schedule 1 and its use is still prohibited under federal law.

So, why is a drug that is still illegal on the federal level getting some traction as a source of medication? What are the arguments for and against medical marijuana?

An edible medical marijuana rice snack labeled and packaged for sale at a medical marijuana dispensary in Sun Valley, California.

MEDICAL MARIJUANA SHOULD BE LEGALIZED THROUGHOUT THE UNITED STATES

The states in which medical marijuana is legal have provided real-world examples of how effective cannabis is for treating certain conditions. "In states in which it's legal, doctors recommend medical marijuana for many conditions and diseases, frequently those that are chronic," writes Jacob Silverman. "Among them are nausea (especially as a result of chemotherapy), loss of appetite, chronic pain, anxiety, arthritis, cancer, AIDS, glaucoma, multiple sclerosis, insomnia, ADHD, epilepsy, inflammation, migraines, and Crohn's disease. The drug is also used to ease pain and improve quality of life for people who are terminally ill."[34]

People in states where medical marijuana is legal generally get a card authorizing them to purchase it with a doctor's recommendation and then go to a special dispensary to get the product. However, because marijuana is still illegal on a federal level, regular pharmacies do not carry the drug, and insurance does not cover the cost of purchasing medicinal marijuana.

Although the FDA, as required by law, continues to tout the dangers of using marijuana and officially denies it has any useful medical application, other government health agencies take a different view. For example, a recent study by the National Institutes of Health noted, "Marijuana is classified by the Drug Enforcement Agency (DEA) as an illegal Schedule I drug which has no accepted medical use.

However, recent studies have shown that medical marijuana is effective in controlling chronic non-cancer pain, alleviating nausea and vomiting associated with chemotherapy, treating wasting syndrome associated with AIDS, and controlling muscle spasms due to multiple sclerosis. These studies state that the alleviating benefits of marijuana outweigh the negative effects of the drug and recommend that marijuana be administered to patients who have failed to respond to other therapies. Despite supporting evidence, the DEA refuses to reclassify marijuana as a Schedule II drug, which would allow physicians to prescribe marijuana to suffering patients."[35]

One of the more exciting areas of research in the use of medical marijuana is as a treatment for Post-Traumatic Stress Disorder. PTSD is a condition suffered by people who have undergone a traumatic event, especially

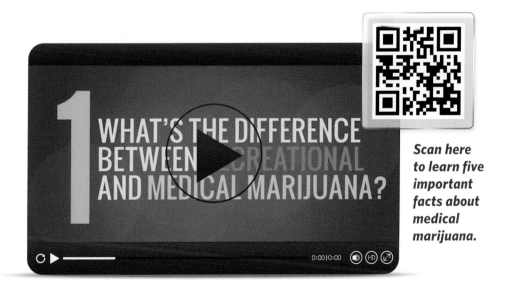

Scan here to learn five important facts about medical marijuana.

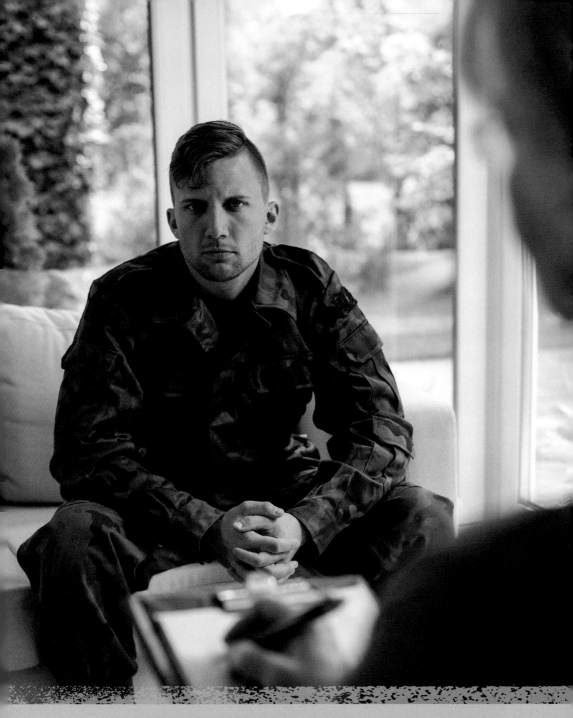

Researchers believe that medical marijuana could be useful in treating psychological problems like post-traumatic stress disorder. However, more study is needed.

soldiers returned from a war zone. The condition can be extremely debilitating if left untreated. People suffering from PTSD often have anxiety attacks, nightmares, and night terrors as a result of what they experienced.

Research in the use of medicinal cannabis for treating PTSD is ongoing. However, the National Institutes of Health notes that "there is a notable lack of large-scale trials, making any final conclusions difficult to confirm at this time."[36]

Most people have heard of the opioid crisis. Opioids are powerful drugs used to treat chronic pain. However, over-prescription of these painkillers has resulted in addiction and even deaths of patients due to overdoses. The Drug Policy Alliance cites a number of studies suggesting that access to legal medicinal marijuana can help to decrease opioid-related deaths by providing an alternative treatment for pain management.

"In states with medical marijuana access, it appears that overdose mortality rates are almost 25 percent lower than in states with no legal access to marijuana, and the reductions in mortality rates strengthened over time," noted a Drug Policy Alliance fact sheet from May 2018. "An analysis of opioid overdose mortality in Colorado including the years prior to and following the legalization of marijuana found that there was a postlegalization reduction of 0.7 deaths per month in the state and that the decades-long upward trend of overdoses trended downwards after 2014."[37]

The fact sheet also noted that legal medical marijuana

has led to a decrease in opioid-related hospitalization and treatment. Drug Policy Alliance found that legal access to medical marijuana resulted in a 23 percent reduction in hospitalizations due to opioid dependence or abuse. "Several studies demonstrate that people who use medical marijuana find that it is a lower-risk alternative to opioids, has fewer harmful side effects, helps manage pain symptoms, lowers likelihood of withdrawal, and is easier to access."[38]

Medical marijuana is in a kind of legal limbo. On the one hand, many states permit and even encourage its use. On the other hand, the federal government still prohibits the use of marijuana, and imposes severe penalties on those convicted of possession or sale of the drug. For the moment, federal authorities have taken a hands-off approach to medical and even recreational marijuana in states that have passed laws allowing them. But a change of policy could mean bad news for anyone who depends on their local dispensary to handle chronic pain or other medical conditions. Considering that medicinal marijuana has been legal for more than twenty years in some states, a sudden federal crackdown would be politically and prac-tically dubious, and would undoubtedly result in political backlash. However, there also seems little prospect of a federal law being passed legalizing medicinal marijuana at this time.

The conflict between federal and state laws concerning the legal use of medical marijuana suggests that making it

> "It doesn't have a high potential for abuse, and there are very legitimate medical applications. In fact, sometimes marijuana is the only thing that works.... It is irresponsible not to provide the best care we can as a medical community, care that could involve marijuana. We have been terribly and systematically misled for nearly seventy years in the United States, and I apologize for my own role in that."[39]
>
> —Dr. Sanjay Gupta, neurosurgeon and medical reporter

legal in all fifty states should be a priority. Federal lawmakers should remove marijuana from Schedule 1 and allow its use on a national level, with safeguards to make certain that its use would be under a doctor's supervision for appropriate medical reasons. Regulations could be enacted that would permit research into additional medicinal applications, with an approval process overseen by the Food and Drug Administration, just like other drugs.

It is worth noting that medical marijuana tends to be lower in THC content than the marijuana sold illegally for recreational use. Some researchers note that the healing effects of medicinal marijuana comes primarily from another substance, called cannabidiol or CBD. "The most well-known ingredient, THC, is responsible for the high that comes from ingesting marijuana, whereas CBD is responsible for many of the healing effects," noted a study in *Psychology Today*. "In fact, multiple studies published in the medical literature suggest that CBD is effective in easing the symptoms of rheumatoid arthritis, anorexia, multiple sclerosis, movement disorders, chronic pain, nausea, neuropathic pain, chemotherapy side effects, and inflammatory bowel disorders."[40]

Many people agree that marijuana is no more dangerous, in and of itself, than alcohol or tobacco—both of which are legal for adults to use. Legalizing medicinal marijuana in all fifty states would permit its full use for treating those chronic conditions for which it has shown effectiveness. Legalization of medical marijuana would make it available for research and development and for training doctors in its clinical uses. Sound regulation would combat abuse and promote the use of cannabis for disease treatment.

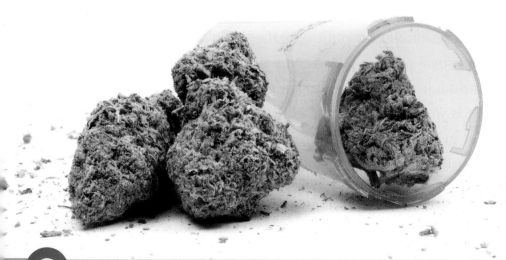

MEDICAL MARIJUANA SHOULD NOT BE LEGALIZED

Arguments against medical marijuana focus on the dangerous nature of the drug. The Center on Addiction takes a dim view of cannabis use under any circumstances, especially by young people:

> Science has proven—and all major scientific and medical organizations agree—that marijuana is both addictive and harmful to the human brain, especially when used as an adolescent. One in every six 16-year-olds who try marijuana will become addicted to it. And if an adolescent has a genetic predisposition for schizophrenia or another psychotic disorder, using marijuana as their brain continues to develop can increase the risk of that disorder.
>
> Marijuana use also has an impact on academic motivation and achievement. Research shows that adolescents who smoke marijuana once a week over a two-year period are almost six times more likely than nonsmokers to drop out of school and over three times less likely to enter college. And scientists have also found that youth marijuana use is associated with lower scores on IQ tests.[41]

In a *Scientific American* article, Roni Jacobson notes that medical marijuana has not been thoroughly tested for both effectiveness and safety. "Despite its surging popularity, the jury is still out on whether marijuana is truly the panacea its supporters claim it to be," Jacobson writes. "Until recently, the drug's illegal status impeded rigorous study of its effectiveness. Several research groups are now taking advantage of today's looser laws to seek out answers."[42]

Many experts say that more research is needed before medical marijuana should be used to treat illnesses. It would be preferable for the Food and Drug Administration to loosen regulations enough to permit clinical trials of

"As a physician I have sympathy for patients suffering from pain and other medical conditions. Although I understand many believe marijuana is the most effective drug in combating their medical ailments, I would caution against this assumption due to the lack of consistent, repeatable scientific data available to prove marijuana's benefits. Based on current evidence, I believe that marijuana is a dangerous drug and that there are less dangerous medicines offering the same relief from pain and other medical symptoms."[43]
—Dr. Bill Frist, surgeon and former US Senator

medical marijuana, but not allow it into a clinical setting until it goes through the FDA approval process, just like any other drug.

The fact is, medical marijuana has a decidedly mixed result when it comes to treating diseases. Marijuana seems to have a beneficial effect on the nausea caused by chemotherapy and increases the appetite of people suffering from cancer. However, other less controversial drugs are even more effective in this regard. Similarly, while medical marijuana does relieve eye pressure caused by glaucoma, a number of other drugs are more effective and longer lasting.

A number of animal studies suggest that THC may inhibit seizures in people suffering from epilepsy. However, human trials are lacking to draw any definitive conclusions. The same is true for its use in helping HIV/AIDS patients to gain wait, or for treating acute pain and inflammation. Thus, more studies are clearly needed before the drug can be approved for use.

Another problem is social, rather than medical. Legalization of marijuana for medical use may be a "slippery slope" that results in the eventual acceptance of recreational marijuana. In March 2018, Utah Governor Gary

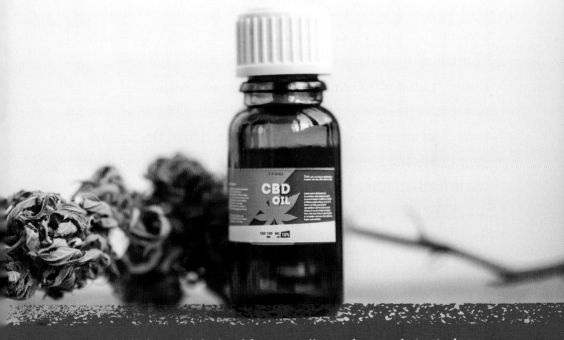

Cannabidiol, an oil derived from marijuana leaves, is touted as a treatment for numerous health conditions. However, there is little hard evidence that it is effective. "Only one purported use for cannabidiol, to treat epilepsy, has significant scientific evidence supporting it," notes health reporter Dennis Thompson.[44]

Herbert pointed this out while opposing a ballot initiative that would make medical marijuana legal in the state. "We need to be cautious as we test and introduce cannabis into our formulary," Herbert said. "I believe the consequences of this initiative, even if they are unintended, will do more harm than good."[45] However, the ballot initiative passed and was signed into law by Herbert in late 2018. The Utah Medical Cannabis Act directs the Utah Department of Health to create a system for the use of medical cannabis cards by March 2020.

Previously, states like Colorado and California first legalized medicinal marijuana, and eventually expanded legalization to recreational forms of the drug. Supporters of medical marijuana consider that process a positive, rather than a problem. However, legal recreational marijuana has not come without problems. These include increased use by young people, a sharp rise in the rate of people driving while under the influence of the drug, and the growth of criminal operations by drug cartels.

There is no reason to legalize medical marijuana until its effects can be thoroughly tested and shown to be more effective than other drugs that aren't accompanied by he same social and economic problems.

TEXT-DEPENDENT QUESTIONS

1. What is THC?
2. What is the FDA's position on medical marijuana?
3. Are there alternatives to medical marijuana for treating nausea and loss of appetite following cancer chemotherapy?

RESEARCH PROJECTS

Find out whether or not medicinal marijuana is legal in your state. If it is legal, ascertain what sort of restrictions the law imposes and what the procedure is for obtaining marijuana to treat a disease. If medicinal marijuana is not legal in your state, find out whether any legislation is proposed or pending. If such legislation exists, write a letter to your state representative explain why you think medicinal marijuana should be made legal or why it should remain illegal, depending on what your beliefs about the issue.

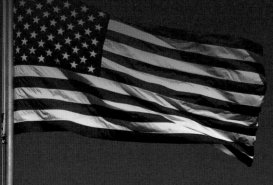

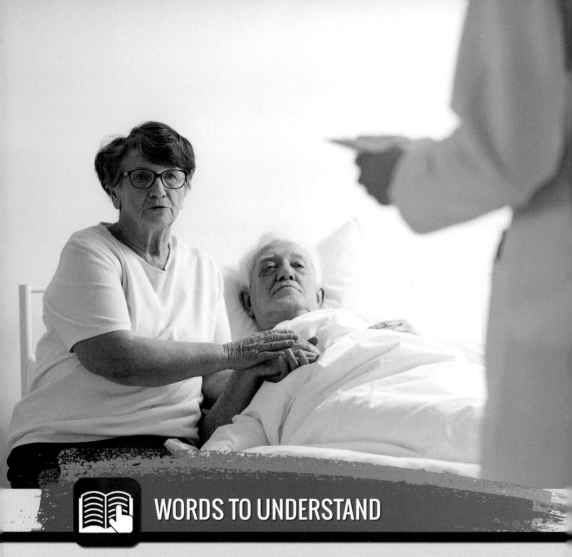

WORDS TO UNDERSTAND

doctor-assisted suicide—the process of ending one's life with the help of a doctor or other medical professional.

euthanasia—having someone kill another human being who is terminally ill or for whom life is not worth living. Often used interchangeably with assisted suicide, but usually undertaken solely by a doctor rather by a patient with the help of one.

palliative care—a program of treatment for patients who have a life-threatening illness, that it meant to reduce their pain and discomfort and improve the quality of their life as much as possible.

SHOULD DOCTOR-ASSISTED SUICIDE BE PERMITTED?

CHAPTER 5

"End-of-life care" is the term used to describe the support and medical care given to a person who is nearing the end of their natural life span. This care does not necessarily happen only in the moments before the person's heart stops beating and their breathing ceases. Older people often live with one or more chronic illnesses. End-of-life care is necessary when there is no longer any possibility of a cure, and it is inevitable that they will succumb.

"At the end of life, each story is different," notes the National Institute on Aging. "Death comes suddenly, or a person lingers, gradually fading. For some older people, the body weakens while the mind stays alert. Others remain physically strong, but cognitive losses take a huge toll. Although everyone dies, each loss is personally felt by those close to the one who has died."[46]

Some people with terminal illness suffer from extreme pain and discomfort. The drugs that help them manage this pain often come with unpleasant side effects. When **palliative care** is no longer sufficient to make a patient comfortable, and there is no possibility of getting better, the patient may prefer to end his or her own life.

CHAPTER 15

"It may seem as though humankind has always opposed medically assisted suicide, but that's actually not true," writes Melanie Radzicki McManus. "In ancient Greece and Rome, there was a fair amount of support for voluntary (and involuntary) 'mercy killings,' particularly to avoid lengthy, painful deaths. Physicians often performed abortions and

DR. DEATH

Dr. Jack Kevorkian (1928–2011) was once one of the most controversial people in America. His public crusade in favor of assisted suicide involved helping terminally ill patients to die even though the practice was not legal. To this end he created a device that he called the Thanatron (Greek for "instrument of death"). When a button was pushed the Thanatron would deliver three doses of fluids: first a saline solution, followed by a painkiller, and finally a fatal dose of the poison potassium chloride.

Kevorkian's first assisted suicide occurred in 1990. The patient, Janet Adkins, was suffering from the early stages of Alzheimer's disease. He met Adkins at a public park in Michigan, and hooked her up to his Thanatron so she could initiate the device. Adkins died within a few minutes. When news of this event occurred, state prosecutors charged Kevorkian with Adkins's murder. The state did not have laws even infanticide, taking the lives of, say, babies born severely disabled. Although the physicians' famed Hippocratic Oath came into prominence in the sixth century BCE—part of which says, 'I will neither give a deadly drug to anybody who asked for it, nor will I make a suggestion to this effect—few doctors of that era followed it to the letter."[47]

Euthanasia occurs when a physician administers a fatal dose of drugs to a sick patient. This is illegal in the United

prohibiting assisted suicide at the time, so the case was dropped. However, Michigan did strip Kevorkian of his license to practice medicine.

Kevorkian soon became a national celebrity, nicknamed "Dr. Death" in the media. Over the next nine years, he found himself in and out of jail for his acts of assisted suicide. Finally, after assisting in the deaths of 130 terminally ill people, the law caught up with Kevorkian. In 1999, he was convicted of second-degree murder in Oakland County, Michigan, and sentenced to twenty-five years in prison.

In 2007, eight years into Kevorkian's sentence, he was released on parole for good behavior. After a tour on the lecture circuit and an HBO movie called *You Don't Know Jack*, the man known as Dr. Death died himself in 2011 from a thrombosis, having suffered for years from hepatitis C, liver cancer, and heart and kidney problems. Kevorkian died naturally without assisted suicide.

States, although it is permitted in some other countries. Euthanasia became legal in Switzerland in 1940. Columbia legalized the practice in 1996, Belgium and the Netherlands in 2002, Luxembourg in 2009, and Great Britain and Canada in 2010.

Doctor-assisted suicide is when a health care professional prescribes or provides the fatal dose, but the patient ingests it himself or herself. During the 1990s, the concept of doctor-assisted suicide gained attention through the work of Dr. Jack Kevorkian. Today, this practice is legal in some US states, including Oregon, Montana, Washington State, Hawaii, Vermont, Colorado, California, and the District of Columbia.

Either way, these are controversial options. The Gallup Organization has found that nearly three-quarters of all Americans support the idea of doctor-assisted suicide. A

Scan here to see Dr. Jack Kevorkian speak about doctor-assisted suicide.

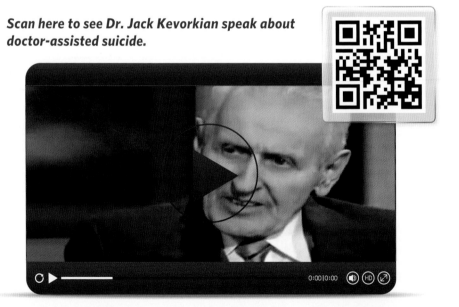

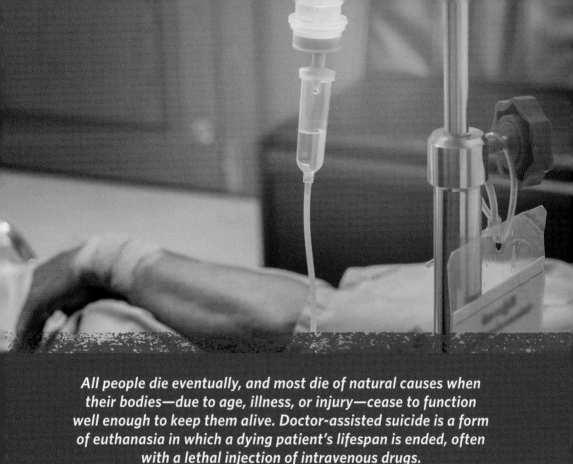

All people die eventually, and most die of natural causes when their bodies—due to age, illness, or injury—cease to function well enough to keep them alive. Doctor-assisted suicide is a form of euthanasia in which a dying patient's lifespan is ended, often with a lethal injection of intravenous drugs.

2018 Gallup Poll found that 72 percent of respondents believe doctors should be legally allowed to end a terminally ill patient's life, using painless methods, if the patient and family request it. However, Gallup found that Americans are more closely divided on the question of whether doctor-assisted suicide is morally permissible, with 54 percent saying the practice is morally acceptable, while 42 percent think doctor-assisted suicide is morally wrong.

The essays that follow provide some of the strongest arguments for and against assisted suicide.

DOCTOR-ASSISTED SUICIDE SHOULD BE AN OPTION

Doctor-assisted suicide should be an option for patients with diseases from which there is no hope of recovery. The slow process of dying can be too much for some people, such as those suffering from cancer. The process is fraught with a great deal of pain, loss of ability to do everyday tasks, and loss of dignity.

The American Cancer Society describes a typical dying process as a result of the disease. Some of the major symptoms include fatigue, pain, loss of appetite, and breathing problems. "Fatigue is the feeling of being tired physically, mentally, and emotionally. Cancer-related fatigue is often defined as an unusual and ongoing sense of extreme tiredness that doesn't get better with rest. Almost everyone with advanced cancer has this symptom."[48]

Pain is the most feared symptom from cancer. "People with cancer often fear pain more than anything else," notes the American Cancer Society. "Pain can make you feel irritable, sleep poorly, decrease your appetite, and decrease your concentration, among many other things."[49]

Loss of appetite is also a feature of dying from cancer. "As time goes on your body may seem to be slowing down. Maybe you're feeling more tired or maybe the pain is getting worse," says the American Cancer Society. "You may become more withdrawn and find yourself eating less and losing weight."[50]

Finally, breathing problems often set in. "Even thinking about breathing problems can be scary. Trouble breathing and/or shortness of breath is very common in people with advanced cancer, but it can be managed at the end of life," the American Cancer Society notes.[51]

Other diseases, such as HIV/AIDS and dementia, also have very unpleasant symptoms as people suffering from them decline. Most people who have terminal illnesses opt for hospice care. Pain and other symptoms can be managed under those conditions. However, some people do not want to go through the indignities and pain of the dying process and would like the option to choose the manner of their deaths when they are still capable of enjoying life.

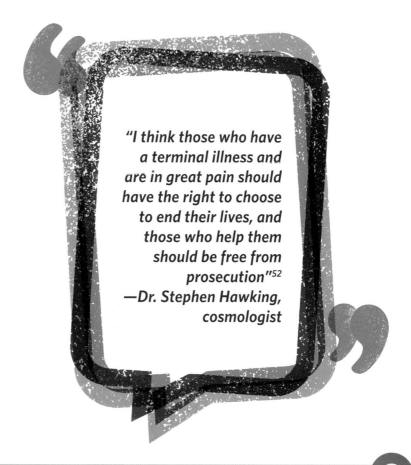

"I think those who have a terminal illness and are in great pain should have the right to choose to end their lives, and those who help them should be free from prosecution"[52]
—Dr. Stephen Hawking, cosmologist

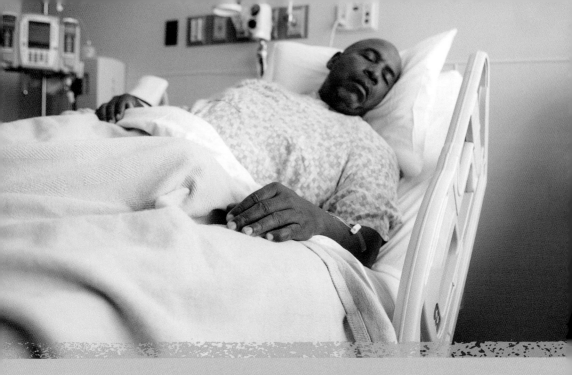

Supporters of doctor-assisted suicide believe that allowing people who are suffering from painful, incurable diseases to "die with dignity" is kinder than forcing them to continue their lives with suffering.

People who make the argument for assisted suicide often point to real-life cases of people who, having grown old and infirm, choose to end their suffering rather than endure further. One of these cases involved an eighty-three-year-old man suffering from severe medical problems that compromised his quality of life.

"Life should have been relatively good for this octogenarian," writes Tarris Rosell, the chair of the Center for Practical Bioethics. "But life was not good. Not anymore. 'My body is all worn out. I'm worn out. Don't want to do this anymore, Doc. They say I can't go home and be safe. And I'm NOT going to a nursing home. No way! Just stop that little gadget that shocks me and the part that keeps my heart going. I want them stopped. Yes, the pacemaker, too. A magnet will stop it, right? Just do it. Please.'"[53]

The gadget in question was a cardiac resynchronization therapy defibrillator (CRT-D) which also included a pacemaker. This man needed both to stay alive. To make a long story short, his doctors acceded to his wishes and turned off the devices. The patient died peacefully, surrounded by his relatives and loved ones.

Sometimes people want assisted suicide when they are not terminally ill, yet their conditions have rendered them incapable of doing anything that would constitute living. Such was the case of a man named Martin, who found himself wishing to die in Great Britain during the years before that country legalized assisted suicide. An article about Martin in the *Guardian* newspaper explained his reasons for seeking physician-assisted suicide:

> Martin is a big man, with once-powerful shoulder muscles and legs. His wife, Felicity, shows pictures of him from three years ago in shorts, sprinting up a Cornish beach with a huge grin on his face.
> "That was days before he had a massive brainstem stroke. Now Martin lies on a hospital-style bed in the converted garage of his home, his large but useless limbs carefully arranged into as dignified and comfortable a position as possible. His back is propped up a little, and a computer screen swings out on a metal arm in front of his face. It is his only means of communication—his lifeline to the world outside his head."[54]

Martin was unable to kill himself because of his paralysis, and his relatives were unwilling to transport him to a country where, at the time, assisted suicide was legal, such as Switzerland. He was caught in a legal catch-22, unable to die but not quite capable of living. He was not terminally ill, but for him life, for all practical purposes, was over.

The core of the argument for assisted suicide stems from the notion that a person owns his or her life. If a person wants to die, he or she should be allowed to. If they are unable to do themselves in, they should have the assistance of a doctor or other health care professional to achieve their desire as quickly and as painlessly as possible.

There are many reasons why patients request help to die. "According to the hospice nurses, the most important reasons for requesting assistance with suicide, among patients who received prescriptions for lethal medications, were a desire to control the circumstances of death, a desire to die at home, the belief that continuing to live was pointless, and being ready to die," writes Dr. Linda Ganzini, a scholar at the Center for Ethics in Health Care. "Depression and other psychiatric disorders, lack of social support, and concern about being a financial drain were, according to nurses, relatively unimportant."[55]

Assisted suicide provides a patient a way out of the dying process that often involves pain, loss of dignity, and loss of, for lack of a better term, the enjoyment of life. The option helps ease the fear of a bleak future, providing a way to go out painlessly, before the dying process robs them of what is worth living. Assisted suicide gives a person his or her control over the manner and time of death. People who choose instead to hang on to as much life as possible, using all the tools of medical science with which to do so, have that option. However, people should be granted a choice without the interference of others, especially governments, who have no appreciation of what they are going through.

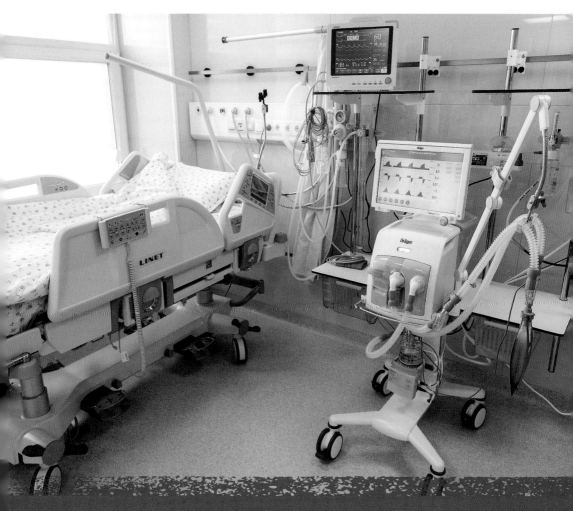

Modern technology, such as this life-support machine, allows us to keep people alive far beyond the time their condition would have killed them in the past.

DOCTOR-ASSISTED SUICIDE SHOULD NOT BE AN OPTION

The Center for Bioethics and Human Dignity takes on the compassion argument for assisted suicide by delving into the case of Sidney Cohen, who was told that he was due to suffer a painful death from cancer in three months.

"The cancer was diagnosed in November, and by January 1 Sidney Cohen described himself as 'bed bound by pain and weakness, having been able to drink only water for six weeks ... desperate, isolated, and frightened' and wishing for euthanasia. If this is what one knows about Sidney Cohen's condition and his feelings about it, does it not seem inhumane to deny him a painless death and, if the prognosis is correct, spare him the suffering he is slated to endure for another month?"[56]

However, that was not the entire story. Eight months after the diagnosis, a still very much alive Mr. Cohen wrote:

> I now know that only death is inevitable, and since coming under the care of the [hospice program] my pain has been relieved completely, my ability to enjoy life restored, and my fears of an agonizing end allayed.... I'm still alive today. My weight and strength have increased since treatment made it possible to eat normally, and I feel that I'm living a full life, worth living. My wife and I have come to accept that I'm dying, and we can now discuss it openly between ourselves and with the [hospice staff], which does much to ease our anxieties.
>   "My experiences have served to convince me that euthanasia, even if voluntary, is fundamentally wrong, and I'm now staunchly against it on religious, moral, intellectual, and spiritual grounds. My wife's views have changed similarly."[57]

The point that Sidney Cohen is trying to make is that he found an alternative to assisted suicide. Even though he was still going to die sooner than most of us, he decided that the option was fundamentally immoral, especially if one could spend one's last days in a modicum of dignity and a lack of pain.

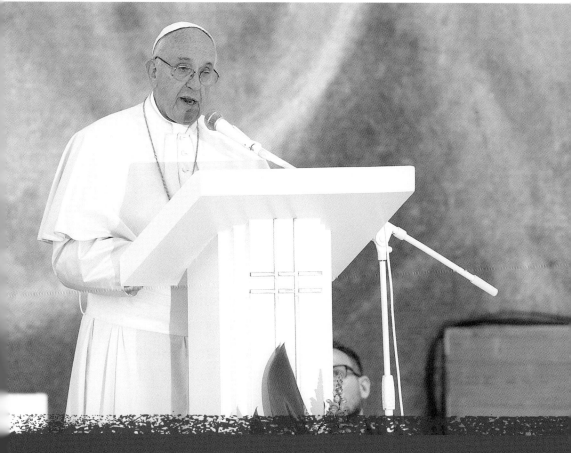

Pope Francis, leader of the Roman Catholic Church, has denounced the right to die movement. The pope has said it is a "false sense of compassion" to consider euthanasia as an act of dignity, because Church teachings regard it as a sin against God and creation.

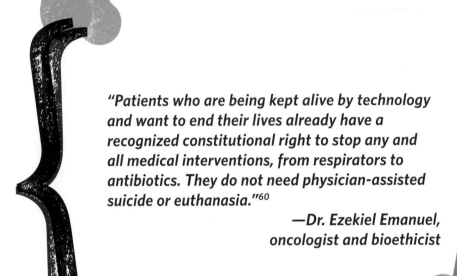

"*Patients who are being kept alive by technology and want to end their lives already have a recognized constitutional right to stop any and all medical interventions, from respirators to antibiotics. They do not need physician-assisted suicide or euthanasia.*"[60]

—Dr. Ezekiel Emanuel, oncologist and bioethicist

The Catholic News Agency, representing the view that all life is sacred, uses the practice of assisted suicide or outright euthanasia in the Netherlands to suggest that legalization is a slippery slope from terminally ill patients choosing the manner of death to doctors picking and choosing who is to die based on their view of whose life is worth living and not necessarily on the patient's desire.

"In the Netherlands, euthanasia has been legally available for decades, and a series of government-ordered surveys have been carried out to track the results. These results are very much more alarming than the optimistic gloss they receive from the survey authors and the Dutch government might suggest. In particular, figures for active non-voluntary life-termination are sometimes as high as 1,000 a year—and this does not include those killed by 'terminal sedation' or palliative drugs given with the explicit purpose of ending life. By no means all of those killed without request non-competent at the time. The survey authors candidly acknowledge that non-voluntary life-termination seems rather difficult to prevent; they suggest that if patients want to live, they should say so clearly, orally and in writing, well in advance."[58]

The United States Conference of Catholic Bishops takes up the theme that assisted suicide can be subject to abuse, especially as a cost-saving measure rather than as an option for people who might choose the manner of their deaths. "Some patients in Oregon and California have received word that their health insurance will pay for assisted suicide but will not pay for treatment that may sustain their lives."[59] In other words, while people could extend their lives, such a treatment would be more expensive than simply ending life quickly and painlessly, making assisted suicide the preferred option whether the patient wanted it or not.

The problem, by the way, is not just one that exists in the United States, Great Britain's Liverpool Care Pathway for the Dying Patient posed similar problems. As the British Journal for General Practice States, "the LCP has come under intense media scrutiny, with the Daily Mail describing it as 'a pathway to euthanasia,' compromising patient autonomy, used to 'free up hospital beds' and even for NHS trusts' financial gain."[61] In other words, patients were being killed by having food and water withdrawn, not because they wished to die, but for morally dubious reasons.

The American Medical Association's view of assisted suicide is uncompromising in its *Journal of Ethics*:

> It is understandable, though tragic, that some patients in extreme duress—such as those suffering from a terminal, painful, debilitating illness—may come to decide that death is preferable to life. However, allowing physicians to participate in assisted suicide would cause more harm than good. Physician-assisted suicide is fundamentally incompatible with the physician's role as healer, would be difficult or impossible to control, and would pose serious societal risks.
>
> Instead of participating in assisted suicide, physicians must aggressively respond to the needs of patients at the end of life. Patients should not be abandoned once it is determined that cure is impossible. Multidisciplinary interventions should be sought including specialty consultation, hospice care, pastoral support, family counseling, and other modalities. Patients near the end of life must continue to receive emotional support, comfort care, adequate pain control, respect for patient autonomy, and good communication.[62]

Those who oppose assisted suicide or euthanasia do so because other, less drastic options exist to manage end-of-life care. The practice could lead from voluntary assisted suicide to doctor-prescribed murder, and having physicians helping people to die compromises their fundamental role as a healer. Assisted suicide is not only wrong on a moral level but is unnecessary.

TEXT-DEPENDENT QUESTIONS

1. What is the difference between euthanasia and doctor-assisted suicide?
2. What was the first country to legalize doctor-assisted suicide in modern times?
3. Why did the Liverpool Care Pathway for the Dying Patient fail?

 RESEARCH PROJECTS

Research what a typical hospice does for a dying patient, including the measures it takes to make him or her comfortable. Delve into the methods the facility may use to prolong life, at least for a little while, if that is what the patient requests.

affidavit—a sworn statement, in writing, that sets out a person's testimony.

affirmative action programs—programs that are intended to improve the educational or employment opportunities of members of minority groups and women.

BCE and CE—alternatives to the traditional Western designation of calendar eras, which used the birth of Jesus as a dividing line. BCE stands for "Before the Common Era," and is equivalent to BC ("Before Christ"). Dates labeled CE, or "Common Era," are equivalent to Anno Domini (AD, or "the Year of Our Lord").

colony—a country or region ruled by another country.

democracy—a country in which the people can vote to choose those who govern them.

discrimination—prejudiced outlook, action, or treatment, often in a negative way.

detention center—a place where people claiming asylum and refugee status are held while their case is investigated.

ethnic cleansing—an attempt to rid a country or region of a particular ethnic group. The term was first used to describe the attempt by Serb nationalists to rid Bosnia of Muslims.

felony—a serious crime; in the United States, a felony is any crime for which the punishment is more than one year in prison or the death penalty.

fundamentalist—beliefs based on a strict biblical or scriptural interpretation of religious law.

median—In statistics, the number that falls in the center of a group, meaning half the numbers are higher than the number and half are lower.

minority—a part of a population different from the majority in some characteristics and often subjected to differential treatment.

paranoia—a mental disorder characterized by the strong belief that the person is being unfairly persecuted.

parole—releasing someone sentenced to prison before the full sentence is served, granted for good behavior.

plaintiff—a person making a complaint in a legal case in civil court.

pro bono—a Latin phrase meaning "for the public good," referring to legal work undertaken without payment or at a reduced fee as a public service.

racial profiling—projecting the characteristics of a few people onto the entire population of a group; for example, when police officers stop people on suspicion of criminal activity solely because of their race.

racism—discrimination against a particular group of people based solely on their racial background.

segregation—the separation or isolation of a race, class, or group from others in society. This can include restricting areas in which members of the race, class, or group can live; placing barriers to social interaction; separate educational facilities; or other discriminatory means.

ORGANIZATIONS TO CONTACT

Centers for Medicare
and Medicaid Services
7500 Security Boulevard
Baltimore, MD 21244
Website: https://www.cms.gov

Death with Dignity
20 SW 6th Avenue, Suite 1220
Portland, OR 97204
Website: www.deathwithdignity.org

Disabled Rights Education
and Defense Fund,
3075 Adeline Street, Suite 210
Berkeley, CA 94703
Phone: (510) 644-2555
Fax: (510) 841-8645
Email: info@dredf.org
Website: https://dredf.org

Drug Policy Alliance,
131 West 33rd Street, 15th Floor
New York, NY 10001
Phone: (212) 613-8020
Fax: (212) 613-8021
Email: nyc@drugpolicy.org
Website: http://www.drugpolicy.org

National Institutes of Health
9000 Rockville Pike
Bethesda, Maryland 20892
Phone: (301) 496-4000
Website: https://www.nih.gov

National Organization for the
Reform of Marijuana Laws
1100 H Street, NW, Suite 830
Washington, DC 20005
Phone: (202) 483-5500
Email: norml@norml.org
Website: https://norml.org

U.S. Department of Health
and Human Services
330 C. Street, SW
Washington, DC 20201
Website: https://www.acf.hhs.gov/ohs

FURTHER READING

Backes, Michael. *Cannabis Pharmacy: The Practical Guide to Medical Marijuana*. New York: Black Dog and Leventhal, 2017.

Gingrich, Newt. *Saving Lives and Saving Money: Transforming Health and Health Care*. Washington, D.C.: The Alexis de Tocqueville Institution, 2003.

Gorsuch, Neil. *The Future of Assisted Suicide and Euthanasia*. Princeton, NJ: Princeton University Press, 2009.

Gruber, Jonathon. *Health Care Reform: What it Is, Why it Is Necessary, How it Works*. New York: Hill and Wang, 2011.

INTERNET RESOURCES

www.heritage.org/health-care-reform
Heritage Foundation is a conservative organization that offers analysis on health care issues from a free market perspective.

www.brookings.edu/center/center-for-health-policy/
The Brookings Center for Health Policy is a progressive organization that offers proposals to change government health care policy.

www.fraserinstitute.org/studies/health-care
The Fraser Institute is a libertarian think-tank based in Canada that offers analyses of that country's health care system.

www.academyhealth.org/blog/2018-09/high-drug-prices-and-promising-policy-proposals-what-evidence-says
Academy Health provides analysis of why drug prices are high, along with promising policy initiatives proposed in various states.

www.washingtonpost.com/news/in-theory/wp/2016/04/29/5-reasons-marijuana-is-not-medicine/?utm_term=.5681558ffe2b
In this Washington Post op-ed, Professor Bertha Madras of Harvard suggests that medical marijuana has dangerous side effects and should not be approved without extensive clinical trials.

www.focusonthefamily.com/socialissues/life-issues/physician-assisted-suicide/reasons-to-oppose-physician-assisted-suicide
Focus on the Family, a pro-life social conservative organization, provides arguments against assisted suicide.

CHAPTER NOTES

1 Stacy Simon, "Facts & Figures 2018: Rate of Deaths from Cancer Continues Decline," American Cancer Society (January 4, 2018). https://www.cancer.org/latest-news/facts-and-figures-2018-rate-of- deaths-from-cancer-continues-decline.html

2 Jacqueline LaPoint, "Healthcare Costs, Affordability a Major Challenge for Patients," *Recycle Intelligence* (August 21, 2018). https://revcycleintelligence.com/news/healthcare-costs-affordability- a-major-challenge-for-patients

3 Valerie Jarrett, quoted in *Politico Interview* (January 25, 2010). https://www.politico.com/story/ 2010/01/politico-interview-valerie-jarrett-031800

4 Edmund Haislmaier and Doug Badger, "How Obamacare Raised Premiums," The Heritage Foundation (March 5, 2018). https://www.heritage.org/health-care-reform/report/how-obamacare-raised- premiums

5 "Five Technology Innovations That Can Be Applied to Healthcare Sector," *CIO Review* (November 13, 2018). https://www.cioreview.com/news/5-technology-innovations-that-can-be-applied-to-healthcare- sector-nid-27453-cid-31.html

6 Arnold Rosoff, "Amazon, AI, and Medical Records: Do the Benefits Outweigh the Risks," The Wharton School of Business (December 7, 2018). http://knowledge.wharton.upenn.edu/article/ amazon-medical-records/

7 Arthur Linuma, "What is Blockchain and What Can Business Benefit From It?," *Forbes* (April 5, 2018). https://www.forbes.com/sites/forbesagencycouncil/2018/04/05/what-is-blockchain-and-what-can- businesses-benefit-from-it/#62636a3c675f

8 Charles Arthur, "Former Apple CEO John Sculley: the future of our healthcare is in the cloud," *The Guardian* (May 16, 2012). https://www.theguardian.com/technology/2012/may/16/john-sculley-cloud- computing-newton

9 "Robotic Surgery," The Mayo Clinic. https://www.mayoclinic.org/tests-procedures/robotic-surgery/ about/pac-20394974

10 Dom Galeon, "There is No Limit to Human Life Extension," *Futurism* (February 8, 2017). https:// futurism.com/there-is-no-limit-to-human-life-extension

11 Dennis Normile, "CRISPR bombshell: Chinese researcher claims to have created gene-edited twins," *Science* (November 28, 2018). https://www.sciencemag.org/news/2018/11/crispr-bombshell-chinese-researcher-claims-have-created-gene-edited-twins

12 "Medicare for All," Senator Bernie Sanders official website. https://berniesanders.com/ medicareforall/

13 Kao-Ping Chua, "The Case for Universal Healthcare," American Medical Students Association (March 2015). https://www.amsa.org/wp-content/uploads/2015/03/CaseForUHC.pdf

14 Kao-Ping Chua, "The Case for Universal Healthcare."

15 Charles Blouhouse, "The Costs of a National Single-Payer Healthcare System," The Mercatus Center at George Mason University (July 30, 2018). https://www.mercatus.org/ publications/federal-fiscal-policy/costs-national-single-payer-healthcare-system

16 Kate Nocera, "Paul: Right to Health Care is Slavery," Politico.com (May 11, 2011). https:// www.politico.com/story/2011/05/paul-right-to-health-care-is-slavery-054769

17 Bacchus Barua and David Jacques, "Comparing Performance of Universal Healthcare Countries, 2018," The Fraser Institute (November 8, 2018). https://www.fraserinstitute.org/studies/comparing- performance-of-universal-health-care-countries-2018

18 Bacchus Barua, "Waiting Your Turn: Wait Times for Healthcare in Canada, 2017," The Fraser Institute (December 7, 2017). https://www.fraserinstitute.org/studies/waiting-your-turn-wait-times- for-health-care-in-canada-2017

19 "Editorial: UK National Health Service—Beyond Repair," *The Lancet Oncology* (March 1, 2018). https://www.thelancet.com/journals/lanonc/article/PIIS1470-2045(18)30134-7/fulltext

20 S. Walker, S. Palmer, and M. Sculpher, "The Role of NICE Technology Appraisal in NHS Rationing," *British Medical Bulletin* (2007). https://www.ncbi.nlm.nih.gov/pubmed/17409119

21 Daniel Knights, Diana Wood, and Stephen Barclay, "The Liverpool Care Pathway for the Dying: What Went Wrong?" *British Journal of General Practice*, Oct 2013, https://www.ncbi.nlm.nih.gov/pmc/articles/ PMC3782767/

22 Danial E. Baker, "High Drug Prices: So Who is to Blame?" *Hospital Pharmacy* 52, no. 1 (January 2017). https://www.ncbi.nlm.nih.gov/pmc/articles/PMC5278914/

23 Sydney Lupkin, "Five Reasons Prescription Drug Prices Are So High In the US," *Time* (August 23, 2016). http://time.com/money/4462919/prescription-drug-prices-too-high/

24 "Drugs from Europe 'safer than getting them in the USA,' Pfizer VP tells US Senate hearing," *The Pharma Letter* (February 28, 2005). https://www.thepharmaletter.com/article/drugs-from-europe- safer-than-getting-them-in-the-usa-pfizer-vp-tells-us-senate-hearing

25 Michael Womow, "Just What the Doctor Ordered: The Case for Drug Price Controls," *Harvard Political Review* (December 2, 2018). http://harvardpolitics.com/united-states/just-what-the-doctor- ordered-the-case-for-drug-price-controls/

26 Wornow, "Just What the Doctor Ordered."

27 Devidas Menon, "Pharmaceutical Cost Control in Canada: Does it Work?" *Health Affairs* 20, no. 3 (May/June 2001). https://www.healthaffairs.org/doi/10.1377/

CHAPTER NOTES

hlthaff.20.3.92

[28] Chris Lo, "Cost Control: Drug Pricing Policies around the World," *Pharmaceutical Technology* (February 12, 2018). https://www.pharmaceutical-technology.com/features/cost-control-drug-pricing- policies-around-world/

[29] Wayne Winegarden, "Pharmaceutical Price Controls Will Not Improve Health Outcomes in Illinois," *Forbes* (May 17, 2018). https://www.forbes.com/sites/econostats/2018/05/17/pharmaceutical-price- controls-will-not-improve-health-care-outcomes-in-illinois/#13ccd0c470d5

[30] Amy Klobuchar, "Let's work with Trump to reduce drug prices," *USA Today* (December 16, 2016). https://www.usatoday.com/story/opinion/2016/12/13/drug-prices-klobuchar-competition-column/ 95307768/

[31] Elizabeth L. Wright, *Pharmaceutical Price Controls: A Prescription for Disaster,* (Washington, DC: Citizens Against Government Waste, 2018). https://www.cagw.org/reporting/pharmaceutical-price-controls

[32] Wright, *Pharmaceutical Price Controls: A Prescription for Disaster.*

[33] Marie Beaugureau, "Here's Why Insulin is So Expensive—and What You Can Do About It," GoodRx.com (February 9m 2018). https://www.goodrx.com/blog/heres-why-insulin-is-so-expensive- and-what-you-can-do-about-it/

[34] Jacob Silverman, "How Medical Marijuana Works," How Stuff Works" (August 11, 2008). https:// science.howstuffworks.com/medical-marijuana.htm

[35] Peter A. Clark, Kevin Capuzzi, and Cameron Fick, "Medical Marijuana: Medical Necessity Versus Political Agenda," *Medical Science Monitor* 17, no. 12 (December 2011). https:// www.ncbi.nlm.nih.gov/pmc/articles/PMC3628147/

[36] Stephanie Yarnell, "The Use of Medicinal Marijuana for Posttraumatic Stress Disorder: A Review of the Current Literature," *The Primary Care Companion for CNS Disorders* 17, no 3 (May 2015). https:// www.ncbi.nlm.nih.gov/pmc/articles/PMC4578915/

[37] "Marijuana and Opioids," fact sheet, The Drug Policy Alliance (May 2018). http:// www.drugpolicy.org/sites/default/files/marijuana-and-opioids_fact_sheet_may-2018_0.pdf

[38] "Marijuana and Opioids," fact sheet, The Drug Policy Alliance.

[39] Sanjay Gupta, "Why I Changed My Mind on Weed," CNN (August 8, 2013). https://www.cnn.com/ 2013/08/08/health/gupta-changed-mind-marijuana/index.html

[40] Ralph Ryback, "Medical Marijuana: The Science Behind THC and CBD," *Psychology Today* (January 19, 2015). https://www.psychologytoday.com/us/blog/the-truisms-wellness/201510/medical- marijuana-the-science-behind-thc-and-cbd

[41] Kevin A. Sabat, "PhD Shares Important Information on Cannabis Legalization," Center on Addiction (June 13, 2017). https://www.centeronaddiction.org/the-buzz-blog/kevin-sabet-phd-shares-important- lessons-cannabis-legalization?gclid=Cj0KCQiAr93gBRDSARIsADvHiOphQmn3cV1dCZ6kMWWYs1kDJG-33jG_HBz_t sRk_MdA3LbWdg3YWI aAjxvEALw_wcB

[42] Roni Jacobson, "Medical Marijuana: How the Evidence Stacks Up," *Scientific American* (April 22, 2018). https://www.scientificamerican.com/article/medical-marijuana-how-the-evidence-stacks-up/

[43] Bill Frist, "Should Marijuana be a Medical Option," letter to ProCon.Org (October 20, 2003). https://medicalmarijuana.procon.org/view.answers.php?questionID=001325

[44] Dennis Thompson, "CBD Oil: All the Rage, But is it Safe and Effective?" WebMD (May 7, 2018). https://www.webmd.com/pain-management/news/20180507/cbd-oil-all-the-rage-but-is-it-safe- effective#1

[45] Terry Hacienda, "Utah Gov. Says Medical Marijuana is a Slippery Slope", The Fresh Toast (March 21, 2018). https://thefreshtoast.com/cannabis/utah-gov-says-medical-marijuana-is-a-slippery-slope/

[46] National Institute on Aging, "What is End of Life Care?" (May 17, 2017). https://www.nia.nih.gov/ health/what-end-life-care

[47] Melanie Radzicki McManus, "How Medically Assisted Suicide Works," How-StuffWorks (March 2, 2016). https://health.howstuffworks.com/mental-health/coping/medically-assisted-suicide.htm

[48] American Cancer Society, "Physical Symptoms in the Last 2 to 3 Months of Life," American Cancer Society (June 8, 2016). https://www.cancer.org/treat-ment/end-of-life-care/nearing-the-end-of-life/ physical-symptoms.html

[49] American Cancer Society, "Physical Symptoms."

[50] American Cancer Society, "Physical Symptoms."

[51] American Cancer Society, "Physical Symptoms."

[52] Stephen Hawking, quoted in "Assisted Suicide Should Be Option For Ter-minally Ill," Reuters (September 17, 2013). https://www.huffingtonpost.com/2013/09/17/stephen-hawking-assisted- suicide-option_n_3940942.html

[53] Tarris Rosell, "Good Death or Assisted Suicide: The Case of Mr. Perry and His Pacemaker," Center for Practical Bioethics (2018). https://www.practicalbio-ethics.org/case-studies-good-death-or-assisted-suicide.html

[54] Sarah Boseley, "Man in Assisted Suicide Case Spells Out Why He Wants To Be Helped to Die," *The Guardian* (August 18, 2011). https://www.theguardian.com/society/2011/aug/18/man-in-assisted- suicide-case

[55] Linda Ganzini et al., "Experiences of Oregon Nurses and Social Workers with

Hospice Patients Who Requested Assistance with Suicide," *New England Journal of Medicine* 347, no 8 (August 22, 2002). https://www.ncbi.nlm.nih.gov/pubmed/12192019

56 Arthur J. Dyck, *Life's Worth: The Case against Assisted Suicide* (Nashville, Tenn.: William B. Eerdmans Publishing, 2002). Excerpt posted at The Center for Bioethics and Human Dignity, https:// cbhd.org/content/lifes-worth-case-against-assisted-suicide

57 Dyck, *Life's Worth: The Case against Assisted Suicide.*

58 Ezekiel J. Emanuel, "Whose Right to Die," *The Atlantic* (March 1997). https://www.theatlantic.com/magazine/archive/1997/03/whose-right-to-die/304641/

59 Helen Watt, "The Case Against Assisted Dying," Catholic News Agency. https:// www.catholicnewsagency.com/resources/life-and-family/euthanasia-and-assisted-suicide/the-case- against-assisted-dying

60 United States Conference of Catholic Bishops, "Top Reasons to Oppose Assisted Suicide." http:// www.usccb.org/about/pro-life-activities/respect-life-program/2017/top-reasons-to-oppose-assisted- suicide.cfm

61 Daniel Knights, Diana Wood, and Stephen Barclay, "The Liverpool Pathway for the Dying: What Went Wrong?" *British Journal of General Practice* (October 2013). https://www.ncbi.nlm.nih.gov/pmc/ articles/PMC3782767/

62 American Medical Association Council on Ethical and Judicial Affairs, "AMA Code of Medical Ethics' Opinions on Physician Participation in Abortion, Assisted Reproduction, and Physician-Assisted Suicide," *AMA Journal of Ethics* (March 2013). https://journalofethics.ama-assn.org/article/ama-code-medical- ethics-opinions-physician-participation-abortion-assisted-reproduction-and/2013-03

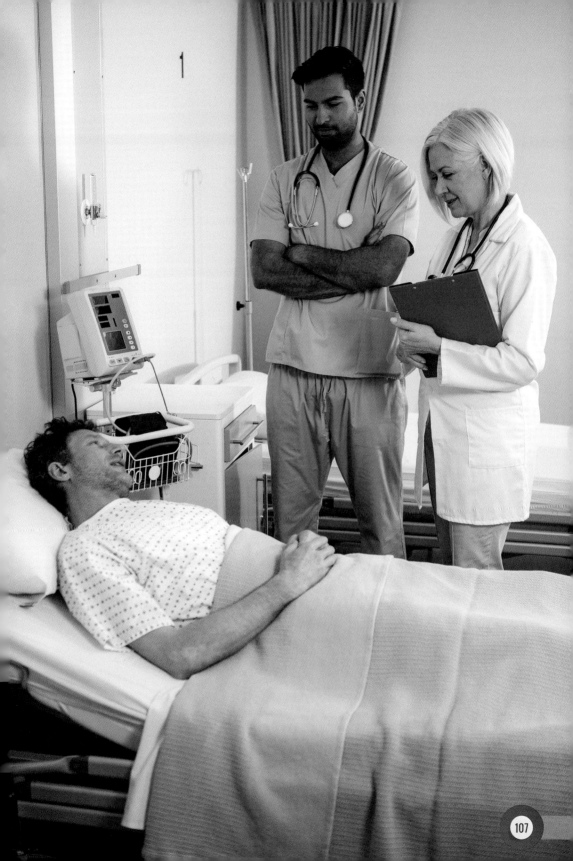

INDEX

INDEX

AUTHOR'S BIOGRAPHY AND CREDITS

ABOUT THE AUTHOR

After working for twenty years as a computer analyst, Mark R. Whittington became a freelance writer. He has worked for Yahoo News and currently writes regularly for The Hill and the Daily Caller on public policy aspects of space exploration. He has been published in the *Wall Street Journal, Forbes, Business Insider, USA Today*, and the *Washington Post*, among other venues.

PICTURE CREDITS